Pam,

Keep moving forward —
that is life's direction.
Welcome the change to
goodness every day.

Doc Marty
10/2013

Mindshift

Mindshift

Your Life Doesn't Have to Suck

BY
DR. MARTY LERMAN, PH.D.
and
DR. SAMUEL Y. KUPPER, PH.D.

authorHOUSE®

AuthorHouse™
1663 Liberty Drive
Bloomington, IN 47403
www.authorhouse.com
Phone: 1-800-839-8640

Published by AuthorHouse   02/06/2013

ISBN: 978-1-4817-1480-8 (sc)
ISBN: 978-1-4817-1479-2 (hc)
ISBN: 978-1-4817-1478-5 (e)

Library of Congress Control Number: 2013902454

CONTENTS

Acknowledgements..vii
Introduction: What Do We Really Know?.........................1

CHAPTER 1:   Fearless Flying 11
CHAPTER 2:   Survivor Against All Odds...........................23
CHAPTER 3:   Helping a Hero...33
CHAPTER 4:   ADHD and *The Force*..................................49
CHAPTER 5:   Discovering Her Sexuality 61
CHAPTER 6:   Childhood Trauma and the Curse......................75
CHAPTER 7:   Permanent Weight Control...........................91
CHAPTER 8:   Driven to Dysfunction................................105
CHAPTER 9:   Look Like a Model.....................................115
CHAPTER 10: Unchartered Waters 125
CHAPTER 11: Childhood Messages....................................135
CHAPTER 12: Unintended Benefits 147
CHAPTER 13: Conclusion 161

About the Authors...165
Resources 167
References..169

ACKNOWLEDGEMENTS

To Dr. Samuel Kupper, I extend my appreciation and gratitude for providing the spark to ignite my writing into action. The transition from wanting to write a book to the actual experience of doing so is beyond description. He shared my want to let people know about what the mind is capable of, and set the creative energy in motion.

To Brandy Lerman, our chief editor and my daughter, my heart-felt thanks. The merging of written thoughts from two people requires an unusual talent and special focus, particularly when blending different writing styles and philosophical thoughts. Your re-writes and suggestions were invaluable.

To Leslie, Michael, Valerie, Dee, Ty, Aryn, John and all my other family and friends for their support, guidance, and patience, I extend a special thank you. To Devin Hastings for his encouragement, listening, mentoring, and friendship, my heart-felt wish for peace and prosperity. To Dr. Mike Stower, my deep appreciation for being there in the early days, when he unrelentingly taught me to stop thinking about hypnosis, and just do it! To Joann Abrahamsen for her wise teachings, and combined with Rebecca Marrs, for teaming up to instill the belief I could master rapid inductions. My friendship and gratitude for a lifetime remains with you both. And finally, to all of my clients from whom I learn, and deeply honor for their courage to face their fears and embrace change.

Doc Marty

INTRODUCTION

What Do We Really Know?

We are consumed by a quest to seek answers for an endless list of questions about our minds and bodies. We are naturally inquisitive, and therefore always pondering the questions of "Why?" and "What do I need to do to fix it?" Yet, when we don't find instant answers within our immediate grasp, we go outside of ourselves to others, willing to try suggestions and remedies that may be more harmful than helpful. You are far more capable of understanding yourself than you think.

What do you really know? Actually! You know much more than your immediate awareness tells you. The knowledge base is housed within the mind. In an awake, conscious state we access a small portion of it. Our ability to think, by using rational and logical thoughts, is how we apply knowledge and solve problems outside of ourselves. Unfortunately, this represents only a fraction of the mind's capacity to relate knowledge. Typically, when we become frustrated or feel dumb, it is the result of not accessing more than that small percentage of knowledge. We know that we know more, even though we can't remember it. "I should be able to figure this out." Then we complain. "Life shouldn't be so hard!" And begin questioning our self-worth. "What is wrong with me?" But the reality is, life doesn't have to suck!

In addition to the problem of accessing inner knowledge, there is also the aggravation of losing motivation and focus. "Why do I start off new projects or a new semester with excitement and determination, and after a while it's so hard to get motivated?" "Why do I want something so badly, but after having it for a while, it's no big deal anymore?" "How did I fall out of love?" "Why did this happen to me?" As hard as we search through our ability to think, the expectation of finding the answers gives way to frustration and negative self-messages of inadequacy. If we really want to be successful, then why do we spend millions of dollars each year attending motivational seminars and still fail to achieve important goals? If we want to overcome bad habits, what stops us? If we want to achieve greater balance in our lives, why do we get so bent out of shape?

The solutions are there, if only we knew how to reach inside our minds to find them. As researchers and philosophers have known for centuries, the mind contains two major parts, the conscious part and the unconscious part. We experience the conscious part when awake. It contains thinking, reasoning, some awareness of long-term and short-term memory, recent feelings, surface understanding of beliefs and attitudes, and some sensory information involving, vision, hearing, smell, taste and touch.

The remainder of the mind's functioning is contained in the unconscious part of the mind. This includes intuition, creativity, imagination, all memory, habits, beliefs, and biological functioning. Its purpose is to keep us in balance and harmony. Our body, mind, and spirit are all interwoven and maintained by the unconscious mind. It is through this matrix of energy that we also experience attraction, bonding, and love.

Sigmund Freud believed the answers to internal questions and conflicts are found in the unconscious, and best understood through dreams. Carl Jung spent years studying cultural symbols and drawings from around the world. It led him to conclude that the unconscious mind is a collective of our current mind, with the accumulated universal experiences of past generations. Albert Einstein understood that we use only a small percentage of our brain in conscious thought. His brilliant awareness of physics came through his creativity and imagination. He was able to naturally access this part of his mind, but never investigated why. The only known bridge into the unconscious mind, while in a wakened state, is with the use of either meditation or hypnosis.

Although meditation and hypnosis might appear similar, they are not. The differences involve their intentions and accessibility. Meditation is a deep state of relaxation in which the thinking part of the mind is put at rest. The goal is the release of negative energy. This is achieved through deep breathing and keeping the conscious mind quiet. It can take considerable time and practice to achieve the meditative state.

Similar to meditation, hypnosis requires the mind and body to relax. Hypnosis has a more positive, results focused orientation. There is usually a desire to change a specific behavior, attitude or belief. It may also be a want to reach a new understanding about a troubling issue or event from the past. Entering the unconscious mind in a hypnotic trance can happen quickly. People can then release negative messages, resolve internal conflicts, find solutions to unhealthy habits, and discover answers to the "Why" and "How" questions.

Hypnosis works as the link to the unconscious mind. We know that hypnosis itself does not cause people to stop smoking, lose weight, eliminate fears, or minimize pain. The unconscious mind actually does the work. As it receives the suggestions, it identifies solutions and moves them into a conscious awareness.

In order for the mind to shift into solution mode and transfer the knowledge to conscious awareness, it has to be free from the influence of negative limiting beliefs. The critical thinking part of the conscious mind, while most helpful in evaluating external information, can be highly resistant to change, even when the change is in our best interest. It can justify or "spin" many harmful outcomes into a distortion of what's real. One common limiting belief is that there is a maximum to the amount of learning and changing we can achieve. It's the idea that you can't teach an old dog new tricks, or the belief, "This is who I am, take it or leave it."

A clear result of clinical hypnosis is that there are no limits to what the human mind can imagine, create, experience, or learn. The answers to all of those questions are found by opening the door to the unconscious mind and experiencing it as it determines what is really possible. The stories of the people within this book began with their decision to open that door. They released negative fears, harmful messages, and limiting beliefs. They discovered hope and the intuitive knowledge that altered their paths, and changed their lives.

Even though all of the stories are different, there are four common features. First, the clients wanted something about their lives to be different. Second, they decided to find the answer to their particular question of "Why." Third, they were willing to experiment with change and try new things in order make their lives better. Lastly, they chose to seek the answers within their own minds after learning about the myths, misconceptions, and misinformation regarding hypnosis.

Without interference from the conscious thinking part of the mind, the rest of the mind opens into a vastness of possibilities and answers. This potential is only bound by the physical restrictions applied to us, and the mental definitions we apply to ourselves. A part of this includes all the influential messages received from parents, siblings, other relatives, friends, religious leaders, teachers, neighbors, and all forms of entertainment and media.

When messages are inconsistent or conflicted, we struggle to maintain balance. These messages create a disturbance generally resulting in some type of bad outcome, most often the use of a negative or soothing habit. The inner conflict experienced when wanting to control weight is a common experience. The desire to eat soothing foods when emotionally upset or stressed can easily overpower the goal to avoid eating unhealthy foods that are high in carbs or sugar. Quite often the choice does not become conscious until after the food is eaten, even though you 'know' you're doing it.

If we know that our unconscious mind influences our conscious behaviors, then why do we not learn to access that part of our mind to make positive and healthy changes in our lives? The answer is that very little attention has been given to teaching children or adults about how to activate and use the unconscious mind. It is not compatible with the repetition and rote memory style of learning taught in public schools. It requires a level of teaching mastery developed over years, and is best applied by trained professionals who teach individual students or small groups. Role-playing and frequent supervised practice are required.

This is one of the two primary reasons few people know about the potential benefits hypnosis can provide. As people discover the positive results, they talk to relatives and friends, who become the next students or clients. The media does not promote hypnosis on a large scale simply because it is a positive experience with almost no negative effects that can be sensationalized. When Olympic swimmers and divers win gold medals and mention using self-hypnosis or guided imagery, there is rarely any media interest. When world class bicycle racers are caught using performance enhancing drugs, the media reaction is quite different.

The second reason is that hypnosis has been totally misunderstood as a direct result of early 20th Century media sensationalizing hypnosis. In the earliest days of film making, when movies contained no sound, the 'Silent Film' dramas typically featured a hero, a heroine, and a villain. The characters were clearly recognized by their costumes, facial expressions, and mannerisms. Movie-house piano music was used to create and enhance emotional reactions and build suspense.

Enter, Dr. Svengali, first introduced in 1923 (Mayo, Director). He was an evil, sinister character brought to the movie screen from a novel, similar to the first film creations of Frankenstein and Dracula. Svengali's unique style was to caste 'hypnotic spells' over his victims, so they were 'under his power.' He would command them to perform various unsavory shameful acts. As the movie industry transformed into "talking" films, the character returned several more times.

At the same time, some performing magicians, very much aware of the Svengali character's popularity, began including hypnosis segments in their stage performances. They carried forward the black cloaked dress style and presented themselves as mysterious and powerful. It had great audience appeal, and over the years many of these entertainers stopped the magic portion of their acts, and referred to themselves as 'Hypnotists.'

Opposite the theatrical attraction, there were many religious leaders who took great offense to the movie and stage presentations of an evil, mind controlling character influencing the public audience. They assumed that the character's inaccurate link between hypnosis and mind control was valid. In their zeal to preach against mind control, and encourage their congregations to boycott the movies, hypnosis was included as part of the evil influence. Nothing could be further from the truth. In hypnosis, you, as the client, are in full control and cannot be made or compelled to do anything contrary to your value system. Mind control is an intentional manipulation to achieve a result not initiated or wanted by the client.

Modern stage hypnotists no longer present themselves in the Svengali image. They focus on the fun and comedy aspects of hypnosis. Their routines can have people clucking like chickens or searching under chairs for their names. The presentations are about sharing a unique, good natured entertaining time by engaging the audience to experience their imaginations in a different way. If you do not want to go on the stage, you are not forced or pressured. Stage hypnotists are trained to select volunteer audience members most likely to become good on-stage participants. Clinical hypnotherapists are trained to determine whether a request for hypnosis from potential clients is appropriate.

The following are real stories of real people. The clients' names and some of their personal information were changed to respect their privacy and confidentiality. They came to see Dr. Lerman wanting to solve a specific problem. Most of the clients considered using hypnosis as a last resort. They did not know they were capable of making changes using their unconscious minds. The majority didn't know they even had an unconscious mind! All of them discovered that by using hypnosis they became stronger, as each experienced profound positive change.

In general, very few clients fall short of success. Some continue practicing self-hypnosis and realize that the skill of entering into trance can lead to further self-discovery, and application to other situations. Others go beyond the initially desired benefit, and discover their life-path toward success, healing, and abundance.

As professionals with strong learning and research backgrounds, we are undeterred in our resolution that hypnosis works. It is not a matter of 'belief'—any more than our conviction that people are capable of changing. Hypnotherapy, as shown in the pages which follow, is capable of a positive impact on the lives of many, many people. Changing your life starts with curiosity. Can you wonder what your life would be like if your worst or most annoying habit didn't exist? If you can imagine it, your unconscious mind can create the solution to make that change. Can you imagine healing from emotional wounds suffered years ago that you've tried so hard to bury, only to feel the pain over and over again? What would your life be like after the wounds were healed and you were free from the hurt? You have within you an unlimited source of knowledge, strength, and ability. Hypnosis is the most powerful tool available that can reach into your unconsciousness and free your mind to experience all that life has to offer. Now is the time to shift your mind.

CHAPTER 1

Fearless Flying

John reluctantly arrived at Dr. Lerman's office to see if he could overcome his fear of flying. This phobia is very common, along with its related fear of not being in control. White-knuckled flyers are found on every flight. There are those who will drive for days rather than board an airplane for a four hour flight. The panic reaction is exacerbated and reinforced every time there is a need to fly. For all the rational arguments presenting safety records and comparisons to automobile driving, the remotest possibility of a plane crash carries a much greater intense emotional reaction.

There is no logical or rational basis for this fear. After decades of commercial flights, it's become common knowledge that flying is technically safer than driving. The qualifications and regular testing of pilots can be rationally discussed. The required inspections of planes as mandated by the Federal Aviation Authority, and the advancements in weather forecasting for flights to avoid unsafe areas, are also rational points. Using conscious thoughts to explain each area of concern about a fear can lead people to the conclusion that the fear is irrational. However, these people continue to believe there is a greater degree of control exercised when driving.

All fears and phobias are the result of negative messages or experiences absorbed into our minds. In addition, judgmental messages are constantly given about subjects like behaving in a certain way or physically looking different, clothing choices, sexuality concerns, voicing opinions, supporting political candidates, and having certain friends. For many, these messages are heard as rigid expectations. A belief of inadequacy can develop, triggering a fear of being controlled.

The assortment of messages, coupled with the anticipation of fear we learn, often become internalized, and influences the choices and decisions we make. While logical thought and supportive assurances may work for some people with mild nervousness or worries, it does not work for those with an obsessive fear, and certainly did not work for John. He knew all of the above, but such facts were not able to alleviate his fear.

John was not consciously aware of why flying was such a fear. He just knew that in order to be successful, it was something he had to overcome. As the owner of a small manufacturing business, John was the primary salesperson responsible for meeting with all potential vendors and customers. Despite a desire to expand the client network, it was restricted by his fear of flying. The business could not grow unless the customer base increased. He had to fly.

The thought of flying stirred up nauseating fear and profound sleep disturbance. John would get so worked up he needed at least two shots of alcohol before boarding, without regard for the time of day. As soon as the flight attendants brought the drink cart through, he would have another drink. His doctor prescribed anti-anxiety and sleep medications. John doubled the dosages. He tried every home remedy suggested to him. Nothing worked.

John's girlfriend suggested he try hypnosis. He initially scoffed at the idea—he was a successful business man and, "damn it," he could solve this problem on his own. His girlfriend described her successful experience nine years earlier. She went to a clinical hypnotist to stop smoking and it worked. She persisted in her pleading, and after several months, he agreed to attend an initial appointment.

Doubtful and skeptical do not begin to describe John's thoughts and expectations of hypnosis. To his credit, he was highly motivated to overcome his fear and seize a wider range of business opportunities. For John, the result was more important than the process. He became very knowledgeable about fears and phobias by spending a considerable amount time on the Internet researching, hoping to find a logical answer. He came to understand that his fear was irrational.

The root cause for John's fear of flying was based on the same conviction driving him to be a successful businessman. He needed to be in control. As a passenger in an airplane he was dependent upon external elements like the pilot, crew, aircraft and weather conditions. John was not in charge.

The issue of external control was exacerbated by the check-in security screening at the airport. It reminded him of the potential terrorist threat, which caused more worry. Then his personal belongings were exposed to total strangers, creating a sense of invasion. Additional, he feared a potential body search, should he be identified for displaying excessive nervousness, which he often did.

The solution to John's problem was to change his focus by reframing the situation. Rather than placing flying in the center of his awareness, he learned to unconsciously shift the frame to concentrate on the expected success of the trip. In trance, John learned to visualize his arrival, the meetings and informal discussions, and how he could achieve his desired results. John's anxiety became incidental by focusing on activities he could control in order to impress the client and secure new business.

For the return flight, he learned how to utilize his creativity to imagine experiencing the beneficial changes the trip would foster for his company. Specific, tangible objectives excited his conscious mind. John's newly developed ability to reframe his situation allowed him to unconsciously release his fear of flying. In order to anchor all of the post-hypnotic suggestions he received, John learned a simple self-triggering signal. It allowed him to relax into a self-hypnotic trance to reinforce his mind with confidence and feelings of expected success.

Three sessions later, the fear was gone—no more panic attacks, no more sleepless nights, and no more need for medications or alcohol. In the process, he not only liberated himself from this fear, but discovered an inner control of strength he did not know existed.

Four months later, John called Dr. Lerman's office to schedule what he labeled as a, "refresher appointment." He explained that he was not having any new or recurring problems, but instead he reported being free from the fear of flying, finding it easy to focus on each trip's goals. John felt pride in his ability to overcome a weakness, and it provided a strong boost to his confidence. He was now flying first class to reinforce his image of being a successful businessman. The physical comfort of stretching out his legs further facilitated his relaxation and self-hypnosis. However, John had flight reservations for his first trip to Europe, and needed extra assurance that he could handle the long flight.

Within moments of sitting down in the office John immediately went into a hypnotic trance. He received the same messaging previously suggested. John came out of trance and shared the experience of seeing himself speaking before all of his employees. He was standing on stage in an auditorium containing more than 500 people. Behind him was a large banner with his company's name. He imagined this trip being so successful that his company grew even faster.

While visualizing the desired positive benefits John's trip to France would produce, he saw a powerful positive outcome. He became the head of a much larger company with hundreds of employees. The experience of hypnotic trance liberates people from critical and pragmatic confines of the conscious mind, allowing imagination and creativity to emerge. The result of practicing self-hypnosis for many months made it quite natural for John's imagination to manifest a long-term positive result with vivid details.

Shortly after returning from his trip, John called the office to share how well the trip went. He established a great business relationship with another company, and toured several manufacturing plants producing products complimentary to his. He felt energized with an exciting abundance of creativity, and plans for the future different from anything he had ever known.

John was no longer the skeptical man who first walked into the office. His fear-limiting perception was gone. The concern was no longer about flying, for he had long ago released it. Now, he wanted to learn how to expand his mastery of self-hypnosis in order to integrate his intuitive knowledge with his imagination and creativity.

Again, he immediately went into trance following a rapid induction technique. There were no suggestions as to what he should specifically experience or which aspects of his subconscious mind he should explore. The hypnotic suggestions were very broadly presented to include messages of business success, abundance, confidence and enriching the lives of others. His subconscious mind took these concepts and shaped them into specific operational lessons.

The hypnotic trance experience involves a total relaxation of the body, a free flowing of creativity and intuitive thought, without the restraints of the conscious mind. In a trance state it is possible to experience and sense things about ourselves; to tap into the full depth of our creativity and imagination. It is similar to the experience of children when they become totally engrossed in watching a movie or reading a captivating book. They become so engaged, so involved, they do not want to leave and come back to conscious reality. However, clients are capable of bringing themselves out of trance on their own, or when given the suggestion to do so.

John visited the office for weekly sessions over the next three weeks. Each time he would quickly enter the trance state and receive suggestions to explore those parts of his unconscious mind containing the awareness and solutions he sought. He learned how to release negative feelings like resentments, repressed anger, and rejection connected to past experiences and relationships. These contained negative energy holding him back from moving forward in both his professional career and personal life. Each time, John was in full control over the length of his trances. It was his choice of when to come back to the conscious state.

The releasing work that John did while in trance was not verbalized out loud. He received no suggestions or clues as to what those negative messages might be. Only John would access his memories and determine which stored messages he would cast out. He was in total control and he learned how to accomplish this experience without any additional coaching.

One morning a little over a year and a half later, he called requesting another refresher session. He was leaving for China in four weeks. This was going to be an important business meeting with enormous opportunities for growth. The flight was going to be the longest he had ever taken. He wanted the session to make sure he could handle such a long flight and adjust well to the time change.

The owners of a large Chinese manufacturing company invited him to spend a week visiting their facilities. They offered to pay all of his expenses. They knew of his company's growth and wanted his input and recommendations related to how they could improve their business operations. The owners also wanted to explore the possibility of a business relationship with John's company in the United States. This appeared to have the potential for him to realize the vision he imagined while in trance almost two years before. He used the trance to channel the excitement into what he called a "calmness of positive focus." The trip was an enormous success!

John continues to come in for annual refresher sessions. During his last session, John reflected back to the initial appointment when he felt skeptical that hypnosis could actually help him. He volunteered that at some level of awareness, he believed he was capable of running more than just a small business. However, he lacked self-confidence and feared becoming successful because he was unsure if he could manage a large company. The conscious and subconscious parts of his mind gave him conflicting messages.

Once John overcame the fear of flying, he realized he could release other negative messages. He also learned to access his creativity and imagination as he became more successful. He was no longer influenced by old imbedded messages regarding his limitations. He embraced his new discoveries and applied them to fuel his conscious mind and his decision-making.

John's company now owns a private jet. He frequently flies to Europe and Asia for both business and pleasure. He recently held a successful company meeting in a large auditorium for all of his employees. There were 600 men and women in attendance, along with hundreds more in France and China watching via Internet telecast.

John's story is real. Sharing histories of clients as their story is one of the most effective methods for communicating and explaining the power of the unconscious mind and the effectiveness of hypnosis. Unlike the use of language, which is a conscious thinking process, the unconscious mind communicates through images and sensing. Sometimes the images may appear in a dream-like state. At other times it may be awareness without words or pictures, similar to sensing that we are being watched or followed.

There are those experiences, emotions, and feelings which are real, but words fail to fully communicate the meaning. Remembering an early childhood experience typically involves some or many senses. Sometimes a sensory experience will bring up an old memory, like smelling a turkey baking connects to the childhood experience of Thanksgiving at Grandma's house. This is very different than trying to use words to describe what happens to a turkey as it bakes.

Children are taught vocabulary words throughout their school years, so they can describe thoughts and relate information to others. Unfortunately, by the end of the second grade, or about the age of eight, the most effective technique for teaching the meaning of words is lost. It is when homeroom teachers stop reading stories to their students, and parents stop reading bedtime stories to their children. The imagination is no longer attached to the understanding of new words.

Now imagine sitting around a bonfire with family and friends. As people tell stories of the past, even stories told many times before, there is a captivating experience as each person's imagination becomes engaged. The qualities of relatedness and connectedness are shared at a much deeper understanding than the definitions of specific words. The word, "red" for example, when used in a story associates to much broader understanding than just a primary color.

Describing how the unconscious mind works from personal experience or learned knowledge is a near impossible task. In order to describe it, the conscious mind must be engaged to access vocabulary. The limitless span of imagination and creativity is restricted to conform within the boundaries of words. Abstract concepts like beauty and love are minimized from their almost limitless experience when logic and reasoning are applied. This is the dilemma in describing the experience of being in a hypnotic trance and adequately explaining the power of the unconscious mind.

Attempting to accurately detail it becomes a rather daunting task because the conscious part of the mind is needed to formulate words that others can understand. The awareness of how restraining the conscious mind is in defining experiential knowledge, such as the awareness of death, creates the image of a most inadequate presentation. Yet, people seem to have a common understanding of beauty, love and death.

As human beings, our understanding of abstract concepts comes from our unconscious awareness. The very process of exploring the unconscious mind leads to an inevitable conclusion that the conscious mind knows very little compared to the unconscious. This is the essence of Robert Cooper's contention that we use only 10 percent of our mind in developing our potential (Cooper 2001, xvi). The unknown and uncertain appears to lead people in one of four directions. They become inspired or curious to discover and explore. They cast negative judgments and attempt to influence others through their rightness. They become fearful and anxious. Or they attempt to live their lives totally within conscious awareness, oblivious to their potential.

Through his writings on the Collective Unconsciousness, Carl Jung (Jung 1968, 6-7) understood the unbounded vastness of the mind, and how it acquires knowledge without personal experience or traditional cognitive learning. Milton Erickson believed the power of the unconscious mind to be so huge that solutions to all questions within each individual are self-contained and accessible (Lankton and Lankton 1983, 8-9). Edgar Cayce was absolutely convinced that people communicate messages without boundaries of sound, time or space (Sugrue 1976, 2). Albert Einstein believed the mind was as infinite as the universe (Einstein 1954, 52).

We also know from research conducted on stroke patients that the mind is capable of amazing adaptation and re-learning. It can bypass areas of the brain thought to exclusively control certain functions of the body, and restore pre-stroke functioning by utilizing other parts of the brain

(Levin 2006, S1). People born unable to see due to blindness develop the ability to see through the use of imagination, and create beautiful expressions of vision (Gallagher 2008, 191). We don't know why this occurs, however, we obviously know the mind adapts far beyond what science can explain based solely on human biology.

From past centuries there are chronicles of spontaneous recovery from various illnesses and medical conditions. Modern science traditionally discounts the validity of these reported recoveries because they result from research that used very basic scientific methods. Yet the reality of these experiences cannot be denied. More and more reported case studies are inspiring empirical research. The power of the mind is far greater than Western Science previously acknowledged.

The story of John, and the others which follow, share the use of hypnotherapy and self-hypnosis to access the unconscious mind, freeing it to work naturally. Hypnosis is not a cure or a panacea. It is a tool—a means of accessing the most powerful part of the mind to affect those positive changes that are most desired.

CHAPTER 2

Survivor Against All Odds

Maria's remarkable story is not about a subconscious message that had a negative impact on her life. Rather it is the inspiring journey of a loving wife and mother who defeated stage-four lymphoma. It is a statement about the power of the unconscious mind to direct healing energy throughout the body.

Maria is a 43-year old woman, married with three daughters. Dr. Lerman previously worked with her youngest daughter who had an intense habit of pulling hair out of her head, eyebrows, and legs. The clinical name for this anxiety condition is trichotillomania. Utilizing hypnotherapy, the daughter learned how to release her fear and anger from parental rejection and the habit disappeared. Having witnessed the successful results achieved with her daughter, Maria scheduled a visit to discuss her own issues.

Maria was diagnosed with advanced lymphoma, which is cancer of the lymph system. The original tumor in her armpit was the largest. The oncologist prescribed a rigorous attack plan involving both chemotherapy and radiation treatments. She came to the office not for her own therapy, but to solicit services for more traditional counseling. She wanted help preparing her husband and daughters for her death. Her physician told her the prognosis for her recovery was not good. He was being honest and truthful with her, knowing that patients at stage four have a very low survival rate. She expected to die. Sooner rather than later, and this loving wife and mother wanted her passing to be as non-traumatizing to her family as possible.

Dr. Lerman graciously accepted the request and agreed to schedule a series of therapy sessions with the family. The conversation turned to how she was coping with the chemotherapy and radiation treatments. The typical reactions for most patients include nausea, extreme fatigue, general body soreness, hair loss and other uncomfortable side effects. As is often reported, she said it was the most horrible experience of her life.

He asked her if she might be interested in learning self-hypnosis to see if it might alleviate some of her discomfort and physical pain. He shared with her several examples of how hypnotherapy is used to alter perception and reduce chronic pain. Knowing how successful hypnosis had been in resolving her daughter's problem, Maria agreed to come in and learn self-hypnosis. As she expressed it, anything that could help her reduce the effect of these treatments would be a welcomed improvement.

In many ways, self-hypnosis is the ultimate tool available for people who feel the need to be in control of themselves, or those afraid of other people controlling them. Even though hypnosis cannot force you to do something against your will, some people are fearful. For most people, their only awareness of hypnosis is the stage hypnotists who entertain people in comedy clubs, on cruise ships, and at charity fundraisers. Others may be opposed to it for religious reasons, even though these reasons are not accurate understandings of hypnosis. While in the trance, your mind is not under another person's control. To the contrary, your intuitive knowledge is at the forefront to protect your mind from intrusive negative suggestions.

In Maria's situation there was no fear of experiencing trance. She simply wanted a tool she could use to minimize the awful side effects of the cancer treatments. She needed to release the mental tension and prolonged fatigue sensation. Teaching Maria self-hypnosis empowered her with a tool she could use as needed.

While in a hypnotic trance at the office, Maria learned how to put herself into trance. She received an auto-hypnotic suggestion which would induce the hypnotic trance through a specific action. More common auto-hypnotic suggestions include rubbing certain fingers together, holding a smooth rock or bead, looking at a picture, or listening to a special piece of music. The most effective are those the client already has a positive connection to, so acceptance level and comfort are established.

The life history Maria provided allowed for the development of a specific hypnotic suggestion that could alleviate or neutralize the nausea associated with the treatments. The goal was to teach her to separate, or detach, the feelings from an event. This would allow the creative part of her unconscious mind, working with her memory to find another, less noxious, association. Maria truly loved her children and she loved every aspect of being pregnant. Even though she experienced morning sickness and nausea during the early part of her first pregnancy, she was so focused on the joy of becoming a mother it was simply a temporary annoyance. During her subsequent pregnancies, she never experienced the nausea or morning sickness. She embraced pregnancy as an overwhelmingly positive and rewarding experience.

Maria was able to form an unconscious association of nausea with a powerfully positive event in her life—pregnancy. Now when she received chemotherapy, rather than feeling nauseous and relating it to the cancer treatment, she instead related the nausea to her initial changes of becoming pregnant. By embracing it as simply an annoyance along the path of experiencing the birth of her first child, it no longer had a debilitating effect on her. This was her first mind shift.

In the succeeding weeks, Maria came into the office to continue refreshing her skills for using self-hypnosis. She was experiencing significantly less pain and discomfort during her radiation and chemotherapy treatments. Her curiosity regarding the power of hypnotic suggestion grew. She wanted to know if hypnosis could help her healing. Based on the results Maria obtained to that point, it seemed like a logical question. However, this is a clear departure point from Western Medical Science. Up until then, all of her progress could be explained as adaptation; perhaps some placebo effect, fueled by her emotional strength and determination. She was not altering the molecular structure of her body or what it contained, at least not intentionally.

We are entering into the realm of both the power of the human unconscious mind as understood by Jung and Erickson, and that of traditional Asian beliefs. People living in western civilization are discovering and beginning to appreciate the concept of Qi, the energy that flows within human beings. The Chinese have long believed that our bodies are composed of more than organs, muscles, tissues, bones, nerves and blood vessels. There is also an inner energy field which circulates within our body. The belief spanning thousands of years throughout China, India and rest of Asia, is that our illnesses are due to the improper balancing of our energy field. When we learn to control or direct this inner energy field, it provides a natural protection and source for healing.

What traditional Asian philosophy and practices refer to as a meditative state is similar to a self-hypnotic trance. Traditional Chinese believe that for those who learn the art of meditation—the skill of entering this inner quiet state, leaving conscious thought behind and focusing inward—the flow of energy can be self-directed. Chinese medicine also believes that by externally applying acupuncture needles energy can be redirected.

In the early 1970s James Reston, a famous writer for the New York Times, received permission from the Chinese government to visit the places where he was stationed 30 years earlier, during World War II. His trip was part of a much larger project which would eventually open trade between the United States and China. While there he was suddenly struck with appendicitis. Emergency surgery was done in Beijing. After the surgery, rather than receiving pain medication, he was treated with acupuncture. It successfully blocked the pain.

The doctor inserted a series of extremely thin needles into Reston's body aligning with the energy channel to stop the flow of energy. The nerve endings surrounding the area where the incision was made stopped sending pain messages to the brain. Reston experienced no pain and no infection (Reston 1971, 1). He wrote highly publicized articles about the experience, and the Western world began to look upon acupuncture in a totally different light. Similar to acupuncture, hypnosis can access the intuitive knowledge that focuses healing energy on the parts of the body in need of healing, as well as pain reduction.

The result of Maria's curiosity led to a series of intensive hypnotherapy sessions. These were designed to engage her unconscious mind to focus on healing while using her Qi to carry the healing where needed. To complement the in-office sessions, she received a CD recording of a session and was instructed to listen to it daily. The positive recorded messages became a daily reinforcement along with her self-hypnosis program. Within two weeks Maria reported beginning to experience an awareness of increased strength and healing. While in trance she reported sensing a resurgence of both mental and physical energy. Her hair loss stopped and the nausea became minimal.

At her next medical exam a month later, she claimed the oncologist was looking at her strangely. When she asked him what was wrong he responded that nothing was wrong. He had simply never seen her smiling before and thought it was rather peculiar, given her diagnosis and chronic complaints about the treatments. He had difficulty finding the tumor by hand examination and ordered an MRI. The tumor was smaller than at her last visit. The oncologist scheduled her in for the next round of chemotherapy.

Maria continued her self-hypnosis program and listened to her CD daily. Six weeks later the oncologist again could not find the tumor by hand massage. A new MRI indicated it had gotten even smaller. The doctor reduced the dosage amount of chemotherapy. He also gave her medical clearance to take the previously planned vacation to Europe with her family that summer. The trip was one of her 'bucket list' items, but now it was shaping up as a celebration experience. Laughter returned to her daily life.

Three months later at her next visit with the oncologist, the tumor was one third of the size from the last MRI. For the first time she shared with the oncologist that her hypnosis sessions were not just helping manage the side effects of treatment, but also included specific messages of restoring her to good health and good spirits. He encouraged her to keep right on doing it, though appearing somewhat skeptical.

Upon her return from Europe, she came to see Dr. Lerman and report on her progress. In addition to having an incredibly wonderful time on vacation, she burst into tears exclaiming she was now symptom free. Her oncologist terminated the radiation treatment schedule. He recommended, and Maria agreed, to one remaining series of chemotherapy before he would downgrade her diagnosis.

Two years after her first session requesting counseling help for her family's grief preparation, Maria was no longer facing a death sentence. Her journey from first receiving the shattering news of the cancer, through the initial treatments, losing her hair, shopping for wigs, receiving amazing care and support from the physicians and nurses at the hospital, re-contacting Dr. Lerman, traveling through Europe, and receiving the remission diagnosis was sent out over the Internet by her sister. Maria became "friends" with thousands of other cancer survivors and family members. She now volunteers time at a cancer treatment facility and helps coordinate 5-K and 10-K events raising funds for cancer research. She is a full-time mom and wife, loving and cherishing every moment

We know the power of the mind can heal. It naturally does this to take care of scratches, cuts, abrasions, muscle injuries, viruses, bacteria, and various other potential threats to our physical health. Part of healing comes from the messaging we receive. As children, when we hear, "it's no big deal," in response to minor injuries and illnesses, we believe the message and the healing naturally happens. Even with broken bones, the cast or sling only immobilizes the arm or leg, the healing happens naturally; and children heal very quickly. Unfortunately, once we move into adulthood we have absorbed many messages conveying themes of tragedy, pronounced pain, and sometimes death.

The same injuries suffered as children become 'awful.' Until recently, it was fairly common for physicians to give terminally-diagnosed patients a prognosis for when to expect death. Not surprisingly, patients quite often fulfilled that expectation—they died when they were supposed to. Physicians believed they were helping their patients by giving them a time frame. We now know from repeated studies that when death is not imminent, the accuracy of these prognoses has enormous variance. When death is predicted to happen outside of six months, there is little validity to assigning a specific number of months (Hagerty, Butow, and others 2005, 1049; Lamont and Christakis 2001, 1104; Hartwell et al 2008, 726).

Unless death is immediately about to occur, illness does not dictate a predictable time for death—it's the message about the illness that creates an expectation of when. This is particularly true when the message comes from those perceived as authority figures, like doctors and parents. By removing the negative messaging, the body's natural healing ability is freely allowed to work. This is not to suggest that all illnesses can be cured simply by giving the subconscious mind messages. However, we now understand that the human mind contains healing capabilities far beyond what medical science was previously willing to accept.

Maria has a somewhat unique story. Note that while Maria utilized hypnotherapy, she continued traditional cancer treatments. Nothing is being suggested that hypnotherapy is a substitute for the treatments prescribed by oncologists.

Changing the flow of inner energy to promote natural healing is not a new concept in America. In 1979 Norman Cousins wrote a book about his own healing experience, Anatomy of an Illness. He described the use of laughter as the key factor in his successful battle against a 'terminal' degenerative connective tissue disease. He lived 20 years longer than several physicians predicted.

Only very recently has the medical profession, beyond the small percentage of homeopathic physicians, begun acknowledging the natural connection between the mind and body. Human beings are comprised of a vast system of interwoven connections linking the mind, the body and the spirit. We are also connected by energy to each other. To only focus attention on one part or one function of the body, while ignoring the rest, reduces our essence to that of mechanical objects. We are not robots, androids, or a medical chart of symptoms.

The mind does influence our physical body. Whether you understand and accept the presence of our inner energy field, it becomes secondary to the healing that occurred in Maria's case. This is not a religious concept or political position that falls into a belief system. It is indisputable that people can use their unconscious mind to empower the body's natural healing process.

CHAPTER 3

Helping a Hero

In recounting the story of Ryan, it is our fervent hope and prayer that the following story can be of assistance to the veterans of our Armed Services, as well as those currently serving. When experiences are so shockingly beyond the mind's ability to process them, the extreme confusion can lead to many negative reactions. There is often a tendency to assign self-blame, as if we should have known better. We then personalize the experience so it becomes a definition of who we are. It is the difference between being victimized by an outside event versus a self-definition of being a victim. This is the lesson learned with Ryan. It is equally applicable to men, women, and children who suffer from Post-traumatic Stress Disorder (PTSD) not military related.

As a society we became intensely aware of PTSD during the Vietnam War as combat veterans returned home. The weapons faced by soldiers were no longer just rifles, machine guns, bayonets and mortar shells, but included bamboo stakes and exploding devices hidden in the clothing and belongings of children and elderly people. Troops faced an unprecedented potential for trauma at the point where the distinction blurred between civilians and enemy forces. There were no front lines and no enemy regiments with whom to engage in conventional warfare.

The Veteran's Administration estimates a significant number of all returning combat soldiers from Iraq and Afghanistan are experiencing mental illness conditions. "As many as 50% of veterans seeking treatment screen positive for PTSD (Ramchand 2010, 59)." Research findings presented to the American Psychiatric Association's 2011 annual meeting indicated almost 20 percent of National Guard women deployed to Iraq in returned home with PTSD (Roan 2011). Between 15 and 30 percent of first-responders to the World Trade Center bombings continued experiencing it ten years after 9/11 (Ochs 2011).

Post-traumatic Stress Disorder is a mental condition which results when people experience an event or series of events so shocking that the mind has no ability to immediately process or release the emotional jolt. The most commonly reported reactions include intense fear and helplessness. People will frequently replay the event over and over in their minds, along with flashbacks, recurring nightmares, hypersensitivity, and avoidance of all situations or activities resembling part of the traumatic experience. There is a tendency to withdraw from family members, refuse to participate in social activities and develop instant anger or anxiety to seemingly mild stress. When the reactions have occurred within four weeks, Acute Stress Disorder can be diagnosed. The expanded diagnosis of Post-traumatic Stress Disorder is applied when symptoms have continued for more than one month (DSM-IV-TR 2000, 463-467).

The intensity of the shock is compounded when several senses are involved. Vision, hearing, smell, taste and touch combine to create a powerful imprint on the unconscious mind. When the sensory awareness operates in an emotionally charged containment of fear, the effect can become long-lasting. Medications for depression and anxiety may help lessen some of the problems for a short time. Supportive group therapy will help some people release parts of the trauma by sharing experiences with others similarly affected. However, the only way to totally stop PTSD symptoms is to detach the emotions from the experience. This is a primary result of hypnotherapy.

Detaching emotions from the events was one of the hardest lessons Ryan ever learned. At 49 years of age, Ryan was a proud Veteran having served 12 years in the Marine Corps, including two tours of duty in the first Gulf War. During his service time he received three medals for bravery and honor, as well as a field promotion to his retiring rank of first sergeant.

Upon return from his second tour in Iraq, Ryan's first wife immediately noticed that he was very different from the man she said goodbye to 12 months earlier. He was sullen, irritable, reclusive and distant from her and their daughter. His dress uniform hung on the inside of the bedroom closet door for months. He was drinking whiskey and chain smoking cigarettes daily, neither of which he did before. She would find him asleep in the middle of the night curled on the floor in the corner of the bedroom. Their love-making was no longer loving. He became very aggressive, almost brutal, and insensitive to her.

Ryan's wife begged him to get help. She made several calls to the local Veterans Affairs (VA) Hospital to get him in for an evaluation. He resisted for many weeks until she threatened to take their daughter and move out. His experience with the VA Hospital was exasperating and extremely frustrating. First, the administration staff could not find his records. After finally locating his records, they discovered an opened, but not closed, "Missing in Action" report. Then, they had to resolve a non-processed order sending him to a military hospital in Frankfurt, Germany. This initial appointment, scheduled six weeks in advance so the hospital staff could secure his records, was put off an additional six weeks so the problems in his records could be corrected.

Upon Ryan's return to the hospital, he fully expected he would be there the better part of the morning. He was not expecting it would take three hours to move from the crowded waiting area to the dressing room, and an additional three hours to receive a medical exam. Then he waited another hour to see the psychiatrist. Had Ryan not originally signed in at 6:45 that morning, he would have been sent home and told to return the next day. The difference between how he was valued while on active duty status versus now was very disheartening. But, he was a Marine, and complaining was not a part of his make-up.

The psychiatric evaluation was very specific, and focused primarily on Ryan's combat experience. He had trouble remembering most of the second tour, particularly the final four months before shipping back home to Texas. At the end of the evaluation, the psychiatrist wrote out a prescription for medications: one to help Ryan sleep, another to lower his anxiety level and a third to balance his thoughts. He also referred him to an out-reach PTSD clinic for group therapy.

Ryan reluctantly took the medications and attended several of the group sessions. He thought most of the men in the group were "pansies" and saw no value talking about his combat experience, especially to guys beneath him in rank. He voiced the complaint to another "shrink" at his eight week follow up session. He was told changes were coming soon to the outreach program. Nothing happened and he stopped attending. Three months later the outreach program closed its doors and no type of counseling services replaced it.

Ryan gained weight and when he discovered this was common for people taking the thought stabilizing medication, he stopped taking it and the weight gain stopped. He also learned the anti-anxiety medication was chemically addicting. This was not something he would allow. He did not perceive his daily alcohol consumption and cigarette smoking as addicting. Ryan read on the Internet how to wean off the medication and did so in four weeks. He liked the sleeping pills because they "knocked me out" and he didn't appear to have any dreams.

The first Fourth of July after discharge triggered the end of Ryan's first marriage. He was still reclusive and wanted no part of huge parties and fireworks. He and his wife planned on camping with another couple at a remote campsite. The children were spending the weekend with friends. As dusk turned to nightfall they sat around a bonfire. First one firecracker went off somewhere in the distance, then another and some in rapid succession. The loudness and frequency increased. Ryan suddenly yelled, "In coming!" and pulled his wife with him to the ground. He then crawled on his belly to their tent, pulled out an assault knife and disappeared into the woods heading toward the direction of the firecrackers.

That was the last time his wife saw Ryan for over four months. There were no phone calls and no messages. A $500 cash advance showed up on the credit card the next day. There were no other money withdrawals and the credit card was not used for any purchases after that one time. The police issued a missing person report, and a returning veterans' outreach support group sent out notices to similar groups around the country. Four months later Ryan was detained in Arlington's National Cemetery by Military Police for being there after hours. All he provided to the MP's were his name, rank and serial number.

Ryan was treated for exposure and malnutrition in a Virginia VA hospital for two days before saying anything more. His wife immediately left her parents' home to be with him. Ryan remained cold and distant. He requested she leave him. He remained in the psychiatric unit of the hospital for four weeks receiving medication and psychotherapy for PTSD.

The day of Ryan's release he applied for re-activation to the Marines. The request was denied. He applied for enlistment into the Coast Guard and received conditional acceptance pending completion of boot camp and psychiatric clearance. He passed both and spent the next three years as a petty officer assigned to a station in Florida. His wife filed for divorce during this time, and he signed all the legal papers without question or protest.

Ryan was shot just days before he was scheduled to take the promotion test for the rank of chief petty officer. His patrol boat was in the process of stopping another boat believed to be smuggling drugs into Florida, when they were fired upon. The crew returned gunfire and the foreign boat exploded and sunk. A bullet entered his side, broke a rib, punctured a lung, and damaged a disk in his spine. There was some nerve damage that affected his left leg, and caused a slight limp, but it was not expected to get any worse over time. His attending nurse, Clara, became a constant companion during his six week stay. They began to develop a personal relationship, and toward the end became lovers.

When Ryan was released from the hospital, he stayed in Clara's apartment and waited word from the Coast Guard concerning his duty status. He received a medical discharge and promptly filed an appeal. His intention was to remain on active duty. The appeal was denied and Ronald fell into a deep depression. She remained with him.

Clara was about to complete her third tour as a Navy nurse. She planned to return to civilian life and continue her nursing career back in her home town just outside of Houston. She invited Ryan to join her and he decided to move with her. He discovered there was a job training program run by a group of veterans, not affiliated with the VA, close to where they would live. He contacted the program and was accepted to participate. His depression had begun to lift and he appeared to handle the move fairly well.

Ryan and Clara married the following spring and she became pregnant a couple months later with their first child. She raised the concern about him not having any contact with his daughter from the first marriage. He had not thought about her in quite a while. After the events of his PTSD mental breakdown in Virginia, he had become so detached from his previous life that it was a mental struggle to re-focus on any part of his first marriage. The last address he had for his ex-wife was in a Houston suburban city about 20 miles away from where he currently lived. He debated in his mind about re-establishing contact and could not reach a decision.

Ryan centered his attention on getting his life moving into a forward direction. He invested a great amount of time at the job training program, and became a staff member. He successfully recruited many businesses to become involved. The training and placement expanded into several different types of job and career opportunities. The media became aware of the program and sent reporters to investigate. One television station decided to run an "in depth" story of the program.

The reporter interviewed the director and several of the participating veterans, including a reluctant, but compliant Ryan. The story was supposed to be about the program, not the individual histories of the people. However, the reporter discovered Ryan's Marine Corps history, including his medal awards. It "added something" to the story, so without Ryan's knowledge or approval, that segment of his life was re-exposed.

The 15-minute feature story aired on a Sunday afternoon. Going beyond the job training program was edited footage of combat scenes from Iraq, along with current footage of Ryan and narration describing, in detail, how he earned his medals and field promotion. Upon seeing this in his living room, he went into shock and the flashbacks and terror shakes began just like it was six years before. Clara had never seen him like this and she became frightened. The last thing he remembered was screaming the word, "No!" He blacked out.

When Ryan regained consciousness, he was in a hospital bed and it was a day and half later. The intensity of the re-trauma, coupled with strong feelings of betrayal, pushed him over the edge. Clara sat with him talking about what happened. When he attempted to leave the bed to use the restroom, he collapsed onto the nightstand. His left leg gave out and would not support him. The doctor came in and ordered an MRI and neurological consult.

The team of physicians was unable to find a physical reason for the neuropathy in Ryan's leg. A psychiatrist met with Ryan, reviewed the medical reports, and talked to Clara. He confirmed the returned PTSD diagnosis, and indicated the leg paralysis was probably a shock reaction re-experiencing to the trauma. The psychiatrist referred Ryan to a contact person at another VA Outreach Center. He left the hospital in a wheelchair.

Clara convinced Ryan to go to at least find out if anything was different from his previous VA experiences. He agreed and met with the program coordinator, a retired Marine Corps chaplain and mental health clinical counselor. Ryan expected he would get directed back into the VA system, which he was prepared to decline. Instead, they talked for several hours, and Ryan felt a connection of trust. He was encouraged to contact an independent mental health provider who worked with PTSD clients, and specialized in hypnotherapy. He and Clara began researching to find out more about the recommended therapist and making phone calls.

Ryan and Dr. Lerman spent about 20 minutes on the phone. Establishing rapport very quickly is a critical necessity for people suffering with prolonged PTSD. The positive referral from the chaplain was extremely helpful. Particularly for a combat veteran, whose adult life was immersed in the military, there is a clear need to demonstrate trust, safety and confidence.

Ryan clearly understood clinical records were kept to a minimum and would not be shared without his written consent. He had the freedom to inspect the records as he chose, and he could record the sessions if he wanted. He was very curious to learn more about hypnotherapy and scheduled the initial appointment.

Ryan and Clara came in together. He did not trust his memory and felt Clara could help answer the kinds of questions always asked at first-time appointments. He wheeled himself into the office, and seeing the sofa jokingly asked if he needed to lie down. Then he asked if he would need to stare at a pocket watch. Somewhat relieved hearing "No" to both questions, unless he would feel more comfortable, he shrugged his shoulders and smiled when presented with the pocket watch. He looked pleased as it went back on the bookshelf. Fulfilling the initial expectation can add credibility for the client and sometimes simply the validated awareness is all that is needed.

Ryan listened attentively to the therapy process of detaching feelings from events, and asked several appropriate questions. He agreed to allow himself to relax, and understood this was an important step for hypnosis, as well as the need to lower his overall stress level. As he followed the directions for breathing deeply, his body became less tense. He continued relaxing for about 10 minutes.

Ryan needed to experience that he was in control of his body, and he received a suggestion to wiggle his right thumb and right big toe at the same time whenever he wanted to experience deep relaxation. He practiced doing this twice and indicated success each time. During the therapy process, this type of ideopathic triggering would become expanded to include the left foot and leg, providing an unconscious awareness the paralysis was no longer needed.

Ryan began feeling better almost immediately. After the first visit, he had no problem asking Clara to remain in the waiting area while he came in for the session. The leg paralysis was the last added aspect to the PTSD, and it would be relatively easier to reverse than the earlier trauma reactions. He went back to the relaxation trigger, and received a series of suggestions that encouraged him to relax deeper, by using the thumb and big toe wiggle. As he demonstrated several times maximizing his control, he received an additional suggestion to wiggling the left thumb and left big toe every other time he moved the right thumb and toe. This would allow him to experience the "deepest relaxation possible." Then the suggestion shifted to alternating right and left sides, then to just the big toes.

Ryan previously received the suggestion that his conscious mind might not know what his unconscious mind was experiencing, and he agreed this was fine. So when he received the instruction to open his eyes while still in trance and observe his left toe moving, it did not startle him. If his unconscious mind wanted to also move his left foot and ankle this would be fine as well. As he watched the foot moving, he received the suggestion his calf muscle could tighten and release, the knee could begin slightly bending and the upper leg muscles could begin flexing, however his unconscious mind decided.

In the process of coming out of trance Ryan received the same suggestion about his conscious mind not always knowing what the unconscious mind was doing, and this would always be a pleasant experience. At some point in the future his conscious mind would learn whatever it needed to learn. Once out of trance, he immediately looked down at his left leg and had a huge smile. He looked up and just nodded his approval.

Ryan arrived at the office the following week standing. He was walking with a cane. His positive energy level was peaking and he was ready to tackle the PTSD events. He came in for weekly sessions over the next two months. Each time he would relax and then drift into trance. He participated in several age regressions to re-experience stubbing a toe, hitting his elbow funny bone, dropping a bowling ball on his foot and getting fingers caught in a closing door. He remembered each experience and quickly separated the physical pain, as well as any connected emotionality like feeling dumb or angry. He was taught a pain numbing technique to release hurt, by creating a mental distortion, so his brain would not process the event through the normal nerve pathways. It is similar to the technique practiced by fire-walkers, or martial art masters who demonstrate breaking bricks. They experience no pain or injury.

Ryan experienced a "Swoosh" technique for wiping out a bad memory, simply by replaying it so many times forward and backward, it lost its emotional energy. The unconscious learning continued. His confidence continued growing as well. He was well into a healing mode and expected the continuation of positive results.

In trance, Ryan would go back to the events like a news reporter to gather the facts, not to re-live the experiences. There is no positive clinical value to having the trauma re-experienced. The emotionality will present itself as if it is still happening. It is the reason the old traditional style of police interrogation of people victimized by sexual assault was rarely effective. The fear of the trauma happening again becomes realized each time the story is re-told. Rather than facts becoming clearer, the fear pushes them farther away from conscious memory.

Ryan practiced age regression several times to report on non-traumatic historical events in his life. He went back and identified a favorite second grade teacher. He reported on his first rollercoaster ride, his first dog, the experience of playing spin-the-bottle, and graduating from Marine Corps boot camp. As his confidence grew the suggestion of events to report on became gradually more emotionally charged. When he went back to his first tour in Iraq, he was prepared to report it, not to re-live it. That period of time contained several upsetting events, but nothing of a traumatic influence.

Ryan's second tour started on an emotional charge. He had begun bonding with his daughter, Casey. She started to walk and talk. She loved Daddy's "horsey back" rides and would give him the most incredible bedtime hugs he could imagine. For all of his training and indoctrination to leave behind family and to only think about them after a mission, it was hard. He also knew about the children of all the men in his company. During free time they talked about home, shared photos and plans for the future.

One week into the second tour, the convoy taking Ryan's company through southern Iraq took incoming rocket fire. A lance corporal died in the truck they rode, and three others received wounds requiring their evacuation. Two of the men were married and the lance corporal had a little boy. It was not the first time he pulled a dog tag off a soldier, but it was the first time he pulled one off a "Daddy." As he reported the event, the sadness was obvious. But it was not sadness for himself. He reported the sadness of the situation.

At the end of each report Ryan released a huge sigh. He received a suggestion to breathe deeply and as he exhaled to allow a wave of relaxation flow through his mind and body causing the images to dissipate back into darkened memory cells. Once completed, he would proceed to report on the next important event. His intuitive understanding defined the importance of events and he learned to trust his intuition. He was not led to remember any specific events or coached as to their value.

As Ryan approached signs of mental exhaustion or appeared to take on an overload of emotion, he received suggestions to leave that time and return back to a quiet, peaceful place. The process involved several well-rehearsed parts, so he could easily adapt to the suggestions. He completed the second tour of duty with a very different perspective. In between the reporting stages, various releasing and letting go techniques became part of the healing process. Numerous imbedded metaphors were woven into short stories as well. The metaphors related to building strength, making the best decisions, accepting progress without perfection, maintaining perspective, and trusting positive beliefs.

When Ryan completed all the reporting, the negative emotions were put into a large imagined gunny sack. The sack was attached to a huge helium balloon. Ryan cut the lines holding it next to him, and watched as it sailed up into the clouds, out of awareness forever. The events remained a part of his history. The negative emotions were released. This part of his mission was done.

The next stage of Ryan's healing involved rebuilding the part of his life he left behind. He re-established contact with his ex-wife, sharing his new understandings and learnings. Over a series of letters and phone conversations, she became receptive to meeting. At the recommendation of Dr. Lerman, he contacted the former Marine Corps chaplain who agreed to work with the couple in opening a new dialog.

He re-united with Casey and they began visiting on a regular basis. Clara remained a strong supporter of Ryan's re-found relationship with his daughter. Casey loved coming over and helping to care for her baby half-sister. Two years later Ryan and Clara had another girl. He completed a college degree in engineering. In addition to developing a career; he continues volunteering time with a returning veteran's advocacy program.

Ryan knew when he returned from his second combat tour that something was wrong. He had no perspective or prior learning to serve as a reference. Within this mental confinement he continued feeling the pain, and all the remedies he tried, failed. Ryan was persistent, and to his credit he never quit searching for answers. He knew there was a powerful source of strength inside he just couldn't seem to find. Once he learned through the hypnotic trance experience how to connect with his unconscious mind, he naturally learned how resolve the mental wounds and release the horrors that were trapped inside.

CHAPTER 4

ADHD and *The Force*

Children are not clones. They mature and develop through stages at different speeds and levels of mastery. Some children are early bloomers. Others are delayed learners or late developers. Some children are more passive, while others are more active or aggressive. Some learn best by reading and listening, others by hands on experience, still others by independent trial and error. Some are quick to learn certain subjects while lagging behind in others. Some are bundles of energy and learning is so exciting there is little self-constraint. Yet many parents, teachers, administrators, and politicians seem fixated on the notion that there is a "normal" standard for all students in each grade level, by which all learning and behavior is assessed.

Compounding the problem is the use of rigid starting dates when children are allowed to begin attending school. Childhood experiences are rarely identical. Some might have gone to pre-school, others have not. Some might come from wealthy families and had a nanny teaching them, others not. Some might have older or younger siblings, others might be only children. Some might have been read to every night, others not. The possible list of variables that account for learning readiness is endless. It is not the purpose of this book to debate the politics of public education. But, it is fair to ask the question of "Why?" Why do we insist on having a standard of "normal," and think that overactive children who are not meeting that standard are in need of treatment or medication?

The Center for Disease Control and Prevention funded a 10-year study between the years of 2002 and 2012, involving over 10,000 children. Of those medicated for Attention Deficit/ Hyperactivity Disorder (ADHD), 39.5% in one group and 28.3% in the second group actually met the definition of ADHD. This would indicate that about two-thirds of all children who received medications for this illness were misdiagnosed (McKeown 2012). In another research study, independent teams from four major universities found that 8.4% of all children born in the month prior to their state's cutoff date for kindergarten eligibility—those typically the youngest and most developmentally immature within a grade—are diagnosed with ADHD. The national average is 5.1% (Elder 2010, 644). Putting children on medication would appear to be intended for regulating classroom behavior, rather than helping students learn.

Even if children are accurately diagnosed, the issue of medication remains a questionable practice. Studies continue to report a lack of evidence to support the long-term use of ADHD medications. A 30-year review of medication studies by McMaster University, sponsored by the U.S. Department of Health and Human Services, found no indication that long term use improves educational goals (Charach 2011). Researchers at Oregon Health & Science University (2011) analyzed 2,287 previous studies. Their meta-analysis found no consistent proof that over time, the medications improved academic performance or social achievements.

Their work also found no evidence to support the safety of children taking the medications over a long period of time. This last point is exceptionally alarming considering there are clear indicators of potential medical risks—a consistent finding for several decades by researchers not affiliated with or paid by pharmaceutical companies (Lobliner 2004; Walker 1998, 247; Breggin 2001, 56; Breggin 2008, 254).

Parents are increasingly concerned and many have opted to seek out alternative methods for helping their children. An obvious alternative is exploring the potential these children have for learning how to activate their unconscious minds to discover adaptive solutions. Jason's mother, Joann, was one such concerned parent who decided to find a non-medicinal remedy for her 10-year old son's struggles with school. After scheduling an initial appointment with Dr. Lerman' office, Joann sent in a complete 10-page report detailing Jason's medical history, school experience, and the medication results for the previous three years.

The report contained a great deal of helpful information, which was further clarified in phone conversations. The suggestion of the ADHD diagnosis was part of a school conference with Jason's parents, second grade homeroom teacher, and guidance counselor. Jason consistently received bad marks for not turning in homework, not completing in-school assignments, not paying attention, and not following directions. He was daydreaming instead of reading, blurting out answers to questions during class discussion without being called upon, and not fully utilizing his above average intellectual abilities.

The school personnel explained to Jason's parents, that it was their experience many students show a marked turnaround when they are put on a "mild dose" of medication to help keep them focused. Wanting the best for their child, and having little knowledge about ADHD, they immediately scheduled an exam with their pediatrician. The doctor completed a brief physical exam and listened attentively while Joann described Jason's school behaviors and the suggestion from his teacher and counselor. Joann received a prescription for the recommended pediatric dosage of Adderall and was asked to bring Jason back in four weeks.

Within days Jason's attention span, focus, and turning in completed assignments increased as the previous distractibility significantly decreased. The doctor dismissed his mother's report of reduced appetite as a minor concession compared to the positive results. He believed Jason's appetite would pick up as he continued adjusting to the medication. After a short time, Jason felt very self-conscious about leaving class early to visit the nurse's office for his afternoon dosage. His peers teased him about being "psycho" and "retarded." Yet, the teacher raved about his academic improvement!

Jason's father was very happy about his son's good grades. However, as Joann continued reading stories about stunted growth in children who took this medication, she became more and more concerned about Jason's lacking appetite. During the school spring break she returned to the pediatrician. Jason weighed six pounds less than at his last visit. Joann requested an alternative medication. Jason was put on Vivance, a newer medication purported to not produce the negative side effects of the earlier medications.

Jason's school performance declined slightly, but his teachers were still pleased, and his eating habits improved. Joann remained concerned because she was now observing a negative edginess in Jason's attitude, and increasing negative interactions with his two younger sisters. The father dismissed these concerns as normal sibling rivalry and "growing pains." The pediatrician suggested the mother could stop giving Jason the medication during the summer and then restart it a week before the new school year began. She followed the recommendation and noticed the "sibling rivalry" stopped, his eating habits greatly improved and he was less easily irritated during the summer months. She also began her own Internet search about ADHD, medications, and alternative therapies.

Upon calling her major medical health insurance company, she received the names of behavioral mental health counselors in her area. She contacted a psychologist and began a regimen of weekly behavioral therapy sessions with Jason. After the eighth session Joann questioned why there was no change in his behavior. She particularly focused on Jason's negative attitude at home and at school, as well as his unusual physical lethargy exhibited every time school resumed on Monday's.

The therapist recommended changing the medication again. Since psychologists cannot prescribe medications, the therapist told Jason's mother of one drug she reported particularly effective with many of her other young clients.

Joann returned to the pediatrician's office. After spending less than ten minutes with the physician's assistant (PA), she left with a new prescription for Concerta without ever seeing the doctor. The dosage level would start at 18 milligrams and progressively increase by 18 milligrams every 30 days, leveling off at 72 milligrams daily. This is the maximum dosage recommended for adults. According to the Physicians' Desk Reference (2012), the recommended dosage for children is 36 to 54 milligrams.

Although Joann continued following the directions from the doctor's office and therapist, her apprehension continued to build. Jason did not reach the 72 mg dosage level. He did however, become less and less compliant and more argumentative. At the family Thanksgiving dinner, Jason defiantly yelled a profanity at his grandfather, something totally out of character. Joann decided to stop the medication and find another therapist. Nothing seemed to be working.

During the holiday weekend Joann's brother asked if she might consider taking Jason to a hypnotherapist. He shared his success overcoming a fear of public speaking by working with a certified hypnotist, as well as a subsequent series of sessions to help him lose 30 pounds. At wits' end, Joann brought Jason in for his initial hypnotherapy session two weeks later.

Jason settled himself into the comfortable "hypnosis" chair. He seemed like a rather likeable pre-adolescent. He was open and remarkably articulate. Physics was his favorite subject, specifically everything about space. His fascination also revealed a high level aptitude and passion for learning. As much as he enjoyed these subjects and science in general, he clearly hated school—almost as much as his hatred for having to take "those stupid medicines."

Generally, children do not like taking medication, especially not in order to function like their peers. Children, just like adults, want to be in control of their own minds. This desire is especially seen in those who struggle with ADHD. Despite the common assumption that this disorder equates with abnormality, the associated symptoms are in fact blatant expressions of control! Children do not exercise enough control when excessively talking, fidgeting, or being inattentive. On the other end of the spectrum, they exercise too much control when acting impulsively, impatiently or demanding. With regard to Jason, his struggles were entirely centered on this concept.

Enthusiasm for space and science allowed Jason to easily engage in conversation about the Star Wars movies. He proudly announced having them all on DVD! His favorites were the original first three episodes. When asked to describe "The Force," he closed his eyes, took a deep breath, and began quoting dialog lines from George Lucas' first movie in the initial trilogy, Star Wars Episode IV: A New Hope (1977).

The conversation taking place was not idle chatter. In the process of the initial conversation, clients will typically provide many suggestions for material to construct metaphors and stories that will captivate the unconscious mind. Jason provided the perfect material for a very powerful metaphor. He would learn to use "The Force" in mastering his ability to focus, concentrate, eliminate distractions, and improve memory. As his success built confidence, his attitude toward life became positive and his need for attention and stimulation became self-manageable.

Jason is typical of most people with ADHD. Their unconscious minds are filled with creative ideas which connect to just about any source of external stimulation. They are intellectually bright with an insatiable need to know why. They have a never ending want to experience whatever they wonder about. With maturity into adulthood, they usually learn how to consciously control this wonder and amazement. However, they may continue to have difficulty staying on task, ignoring distractions, following directions and completing assignments.

Young children do not have this control mechanism yet. It is part of social learning acquired through observation and role modeling, as well as interactions in families, pre-school, and early grade school. When social learning is limited, conscious control may be impaired or severely lacking. The goal of hypnosis is to restore the mind's natural process of control, including intuitive curiosity. It allows clients to focus on a specific issue or task while filtering out irrelevant distractions.

Drawing upon Jason's fascination with Star Wars, the metaphor of Luke learning to harness the power of The Force was a fun learning tool. In the film, Obi-Wan blindfolds Luke to teach him how to sense when a zapping orb was about to send out an electric shock. Mastering the anticipation allowed Luke to make adjustments, prior to the shocking pulse, rather than reacting after feeling it. Luke had to trust his intuitive knowledge to focus, concentrate, anticipate, and move. The light saber symbolizes how the conscious mind can become laser focused and extraordinarily accurate by trusting the mind's knowledge.

Embedded within all three movies of the initial Star Wars trilogy, Luke hears the messages, "Concentrate" and "Use The Force" in the voices of Obi-Wan and Yoda. These simple reminders triggered an immediate connection to his mental training in becoming a Jedi Warrior. The effect is similar to how a post-hypnotic suggestion anchors a connection to the unconscious mind. If the sight of your boss creates an instant negative reaction, and you are concerned your attitude may get you in trouble, try picking out one specific flaw in his or her face. Every time you see it, imagine the same flaw on the face of Dumbo or Scooby-Doo or another absurdly looking cartoon face. This is a conscious anchor. Learning connections like this while in a trance state makes them more powerful, and ensures a smiling reaction every time.

Just as Luke learned an anchor, so did Jason. During the hypnosis sessions he learned several clinical anchors. With daily practice he could quickly put himself into a self-hypnotic trance whenever he sensed feeling stressed or distracted. The trance would last for three to four seconds, just long enough for Jason to regain the confidence of knowing he was in control. His favorite anchor was the whistle sound from R2D2 acknowledging agreement. He learned to perfectly imitate it the first time he saw the movie, and repeated it so often he could hear it from memory without having to actually whistle.

Jason became very productive completing assignments and tasks. It was part of his mission and training in becoming a "warrior." As he began to consistently prove how focused he could become, he then learned how to keep his feelings balanced—just like Luke using The Force to keep his anger channeled. His victories elevated his self-esteem as his confidence blossomed. He started having fun playing mental games with himself as he mastered different tasks. He was smiling on his way out the door to school.

Two months after the initial visit, Jason's medication dosage was down to 18 milligrams a day with no negative side effects. His father nicknamed him "Luke," which was how he introduced himself to his new soccer team that spring. During a follow-up phone call with Joann four months later, she reported Jason was completely off medication and doing quite well. He was free of all the previous ADHD symptoms, on the honor roll, and getting along very well with his sisters. Jason finished the entire season on the soccer team, without wanting to quit or throwing a fit about going to practice. It was the first time in four years, since he began participating on team activities that he sustained interest in the activity from its start through completion.

Children of course want to play and have fun, and at times require re-direction. They also want to learn and master activities and concepts. The feelings of pride and confidence from working hard and experiencing success are universal to humans, regardless of age. For people with ADHD there is an internal misdirection creating a blockade. It is most important for parents to know there is an alternative path to provide their children with balance and focus, besides dependency on medications that have unpredictable side effects. Hypnosis reaches the inner understandings of the mind allowing people to release the blockage. Reducing family stress is critical—hope is priceless.

CHAPTER 5

Discovering Her Sexuality

Imagine living with chronic lower pelvic pain and not being able to learn its cause. Imagine being married for almost 17 years and believing that sex without orgasm was the norm for women. Imagine not having any sexual desires or interests. That was the life Kim was living. She changed as a result of self-discovery through the process of hypnosis. She learned to experience the joy and ecstasy of being a sensual woman. Kim has much in common with many women whose beliefs about sex are conditioned by generations of misinformation, passed on by mothers, fathers, older siblings, media, peers, schools, and religious institutions.

Kim was a 36 year old, married mother of two referred by her obstetrician/gynecologist (OB/GYN). In response to some gentle questioning, she confided in him that she did not find sex enjoyable. Other than wanting to conceive her children and satisfy her husband's needs, she had no interest in sex. She had not experienced an orgasm since the onset of a constant pain in her lower pelvic area. Her doctor assured her that he would do everything medically possible to discover the cause of the problem and treat it.

Chronic Pelvic Pain Distress is a very painful illness that can be caused by multiple medical conditions. Kim's OB/GYN understood the symptoms, but could find no cause for them.

There were no signs of infection or endometriosis, no unusual inflammation, no cysts, no cancer, no vascular problems, and no history of physical trauma. Ultrasounds followed by two laparoscopies revealed nothing unusual. Her menstruation cycles were fairly normal and she had not experienced any problems with either pregnancy. The physician assumed Kim's lack of libido was a natural result of the chronic pain.

The OB/GYN referred her to specialists. Each of these doctors ran more tests, performed examinations and could not identify a cause. The last one suggested the problem might be psychogenic, meaning her mind created the medical condition. That physician gave her pain medication and a trial dosage of an anti-depressant medication also designed to reduce pain. The pain decreased, but never completely stopped. Kim was very concerned about the potential side-effects of, and addiction to pain medications.

After 14 months of inconclusive tests, trials of various pain medications, anti-depressants, and more medical consultations, her original OB/GYN suggested she consult with a psychiatrist. According to Kim the psychiatrist did not obtain any social or medical history regarding past trauma, or attempt to determine if there was an underlying psychological factor involved. She was incredulous that the psychiatrist spent less than 15 minutes interviewing her and so quickly agreed with the psychogenic theory. He gave her a prescription for the same anti-depressant she was taking, but doubled the dosage.

After Kim started taking the increased anti-depressant dosage, she plunged into a very depressed state. She experienced occasional thoughts that perhaps her family might be better off without her. For Kim, feeling like a burden on her family was unacceptable. A couple weeks later while watching television with her husband, she saw a commercial for the medication she was taking. The advertisement concluded with a voice quickly rattling off the list of potential side effects. The phrases, "deepening depression," and "suicidal thoughts," sent off alarm bells. Kim let out a loud scream startling her half-asleep husband. Terrified and enraged, she immediately decided to stop taking this drug and find an alternative course of treatment.

The next morning, Kim began an Internet search and discovered references for hypnotherapy. She called her OB/GYN and asked him for a referral. Fortunately, he was also a certified sex educator and familiar with Dr. Lerman's work. Kim scheduled her initial appointment for later that week.

The most obvious question during an initial session for pain management is, "When did you first start feeling this pain?" Kim was 19 years old when it started. We know pain is a reaction to something already experienced, either physical or mental. When asked what happened to her during the year before the pain started, she looked confused. Kim's comments about her life had been exclusively focused on her roles as a wife and mother, not from anything before. It was almost as if she viewed her marriage as the starting point of her life. When she heard the question a second time, her facial expression shifted from one of confusion and curiosity to one of hurt and sadness. With a monotonous tone of voice, she disclosed that her first fiancé, Trey, died one year prior to the onset of her pelvic pain.

Kim and Trey were high school sweethearts, but chose to abstain from sexual activity until they married. Purity and chastity were always values she held. They were reinforced by regular participation in Sunday school at a fundamentalist church that she attended with her family as a child. During adolescence there was an implicit message among the private school students, "a good girl was a virgin until her marriage, and she only had intercourse with her husband to have children and as part of her wifely duties."

Shortly after graduation Trey enlisted in the Marines. He formally proposed marriage to Kim the day before heading to boot camp, and she heartily accepted. After completing boot camp, he received leave until having to report to his base assignment. During this time, the first Gulf War erupted. On the last night of Trey's leave, they could no longer restrain their love, passion or desire. They had sex. It was beautiful, fulfilling, and Kim experienced her first orgasm. Unfortunately, that was the last time she saw Trey. Three weeks later he was killed in a helicopter crash during a training exercise.

Kim shared with Dr. Lerman about feeling intense grief for a long time following the accident. She was distraught and inconsolable while grieving, but her parents and friends remained supportive. About nine months after Trey's death, at the encouragement of her parents, she began socializing and meeting other young adults. Kim was adjusting, or so she thought. It never occurred to her that there was any connection between the onset of her chronic pelvic pain, and the one-year anniversary of Trey's death. Anniversary dates of all kinds are important in our lives, but particularly those marking a loved one's death.

There are often traditions we observe on the anniversaries of days when loved ones died. They help relieve our grief, and allow us to process our emotions with support from family and friends. Often times, we're able to cherish our more positive memories, and move on. Sometimes though, we harbor negative experiences and drag them with us after losing loved ones. We do this for a number of reasons, but the effect is that we never completely let go. As much as we try to bury the negative emotions, they're never far below the surface, and they have a nasty proclivity for affecting biological functioning. This association is part of the mind/body connection.

The obvious relationship to Dr. Lerman between the first year anniversary of her fiancé's death and the onset of Kim's pelvic pain was mentioned, but not pressed. She wasn't ready to understand the connection. Her conscious mind already constructed an alternative and rather firm belief system concerning the events of her life. It would be counter-productive to raise it at this point. Her unconscious mind would revisit this particular mind/body connection after the internal healing had begun.

Kim came into the office for the initial visit with her husband, Darren. He expressed concern about her chronic pelvic pain and wanted to be supportive. He knew about her previous engagement and the fiancé's tragic death, but none of the details leading up to it. Kim's goals for hypnotherapy were to resolve the pain and establish feelings of sexual desire for her husband. She intuitively connected the two without a conscious awareness they were interrelated.

As Kim continued describing the reasons for her visit, she stated she had never experienced an orgasm with her husband. Darren looked astonished and commented on his opinion that they had a good, but not great sex life. His only complaint is that he wanted sexual intimacy with her more than just on Saturday nights. As she fought back tears, she explained she faked the orgasms wanting Darren to feel he was satisfying her.

Kim's emotional distress was further complicated by having to double up on her pain medication every Saturday, while drinking large quantities of wine. Despite these violations of her value system, she allowed the weekly sex and bore the physical pain because she believed it was her duty to keep her husband satisfied. Her longtime belief system remained strong, and empowered her life mission to create a happy home built with a positive and healthy family life.

When one partner is experiencing a sexual problem it is often beneficial to involve the other partner in joint therapy. Due to the strong emotional connections placed upon sexuality and sexual performance, it is very common for the partner of the person experiencing a problem to internalize fault, or feelings of inadequacy. It is also common for the partner to assign blame, anger and rejection when expectations are not fulfilled.

Male egos that are bruised from sexual conflicts are usually the more difficult ones to accept healing and forgiveness.

Kim loved her husband and looked forward to sexually intimate times with him, in spite of the physical pain. They fostered emotional closeness and shared affection, though she never expected to have an orgasm. Once Darren understood her sexuality issues were not because of him, he became even more supportive and encouraging. Both of them were motivated to find a solution that fit within their value system.

Initially, the concept of hypnosis presented a value system challenge for Kim. Her church teachings included a strong prohibition against activities believed to weaken the mind's ability to ward off evil control. Unfortunately, many people uneducated about the reality of hypnosis perpetuate the myth that hypnosis is a form of mind control, when the opposite is actually the truth. It strengthens the mind by promoting balance, harmony and healing. Intuitive knowledge becomes accessible to the conscious mind, thus eliminating self-doubt and emotional and spiritual vulnerability. Kim was advised of the truth behind this, and many other myths surrounding hypnosis. She was also encouraged to record the sessions, and share them with her minister should she choose to do so.

Following Trey's death, Kim unconsciously replaced her positive sexual experience with a punishing negative response. She lost touch with herself and who she was as a woman. The pleasure/pain principle of the human brain is a relatively simple concept to understand. We strive to experience those activities most likely to result in pleasure, while avoiding those things most likely to result in pain. However, when we experience an activity amazingly pleasurable and then are suddenly thrown into a pain-reactive mode of horrifying proportions, the mind is not capable of immediately switching gears. The result is known as shock.

Regardless of whether it is physical shock like soldiers can experience in combat or emotional trauma, shock is the brain's way of shouting, "Stop! No More!" Depending on the intensity of the perceived trauma, people sometimes pass out, potentially experiencing a comma state. Sometimes they overload their denial system, pretending they are all right, only to later experience delayed reactions commonly referred to as Post-traumatic Stress Disorder (PTSD). On more rare occasions, in response to severe perceptions, people disassociate from parts of their mind or body.

The source of Kim's intense pleasure came from the emotional build up with her fiancé, as he was about to go to war. This coupled with the physical pleasure of sexual intercourse and orgasm as she released her virginity. When he suddenly died three weeks later, the pain was so intense her mind was not capable of accepting it. As she grieved the loss in the months following the accident, she began internalizing overwhelming feelings of guilt.

Given her strong religious beliefs and vow of chastity, Kim feared their one moment of passionate weakness had evoked the wrath of God. Perhaps, like Adam and Eve, she caused Trey the loss of his innocence. It created such a distraction that he was unable to respond to that crisis situation costing him his life. Due to the pleasure she experienced, was she now condemned to never experience it again. She would fulfill her ordained purpose in life to marry, honor her husband, and produce children. She should have no expectation of ever having an orgasmic sexual relationship again. These were the powerful internal messages Kim created and maintained.

In order to help Kim let go of the pain, she needed to regain her strength and self-confidence. With these restored, she could then learn to release her subconscious beliefs. The metaphor of traveling through a forest is a symbol for life's journey. It is particularly effective for people who feel lost inside, and are fearful of what lies ahead. The imagination is rich in its ability to picture a vast array of sights, sounds, smells, tastes, and skin reactions. In trance, Kim began to experience the beauty of the forest, to see and touch the trees and flowers, listen to the birds and crickets, and breathe in the clean pure air.

Kim began to welcome her times in the forest. Her initial perception of the forest as a negative scary place changed into a safe place of adventure and discovery. She learned to trust her sense of direction, to know that if she moved in a northerly direction, she could always find her way out of the forest. Her sense of self-confidence grew. Her powers of imagination and creativity grew. Her senses became alive. She was able to reach out and touch, smell, and enjoy all that surrounded her without the past fear.

The next step was to use other imagery to help Kim find those messages and feelings in her unconscious mind. She now knew how to enter a self-hypnotic trance, and visited the forest at home in between her sessions. The forest metaphor expanded. As she reached a part of the forest never before explored, she became aware that it faced a beautiful mountain with a path she could follow taking her to the top. Encouraged to follow the path, she paused to listen to the sounds of the bubbling brook at the bottom of a waterfall, to marvel at the colorful flowers growing alongside the path, to see a mother doe and her newborn fawn calmly and peacefully accept her presence. She felt herself relaxing even deeper into trance. She reached the top of the path and stepped onto a beautiful plateau. She looked skyward at the puffy clouds, the clear blue sky and snow-capped mountains off in the distance.

At the back edge of the plateau she discovered the downside of the mountain was very dark, nothing grew on this side. The sun did not shine there. It was jagged rock as far down as she could see. Scattered near her feet were a variety of dark colored rocks. Each rock belonged to her and contained negative beliefs, actions and feeling from her past. Standing firmly by the side of the cliff with her feet solidly anchored, she threw these rocks one by one over the side of the cliff, listening to them thump and clang off the face of the cliff into the abyss below. She was releasing and cleansing her mind of the negative energy acquired over time preventing her from experiencing life to its fullest.

Kim's homework assignment was to revisit the forest and mountaintop every day. She was free to throw any additional rocks over the edge as her intuition directed. At her next session she reported feeling lighter, less troubled, and a noticeably decreased pain in her pelvic area. Now, she was excited to return to the mountaintop to discover more new learning. This time after casting more stones over the side of the cliff, she went to the center of the plateau and experienced a place of incredible loving and healing warmth. The ground contained many clear crystal stones of varying shapes and sizes. Kim's assignment was to use the stones to create a monument of her testament to her goodness and self-acceptance of her spirituality. Each stone represented a positive feeling, accomplishment, experience, relationship or memory in her life. Having released the negative influences through her imagination and creativity, her unconscious mind rejuvenated positive energy for her to move forward, allowing the restoration of her faith.

The following week she reported visiting the plateau several times. She spent most of her time in the center area, picking up one or two stones each time and adding them to her monument. She was totally comfortable verbalizing what she was doing and describing additions to the monument. During one of the visits she found a small rose colored quartz rock among the new white stones. As she rubbed the stone in her hands she began feeling a warm pleasant sensation in her pelvic area. Later that night she reported having a dream making love with her husband. There was no pain. It was warm, sensual, loving and she reached a climax. The rose quartz rock was in her hand. It was the first erotic dream Kim had since the death of her fiancé.

At Kim's request she received a recommended reading list of books intended to help fill in her sexual knowledge. The list included both fiction and non-fiction. Her two favorite books were Delta of Venus by Anais Nin and Lady Chatterley's

Lover by D. H. Lawrence. She also began renting R-rated and unrated European movies containing scenes of positive sexual intimacy between lovers. Despite her husband's curiosity, she was not yet ready to include him in her new learning. She continued practicing self-hypnosis on a daily basis.

Her sexuality continued developing. Her choice of clothes became more stylish and more revealing when out on dates with Darrin. Her anniversary card to him three weeks later was filled with suggestive sexual messages. She reported putting herself into a trance one evening while stroking the neck of a glass bottle sitting alone in the living room. She became aware of a rather strong sexual desire that brought her out of the trance, but led to a very pleasurable intimate time with her husband when he returned home a short while later.

The rose quartz rock remained a strong symbol for her. While roaming through a flea market with her daughters, she came across a table display of various rocks and different colored quartz crystals. She found a rose colored rock just like she imagined. She had it mounted onto a necklace and wears it whenever the mood strikes her. Kim also discovered the mental ability to create the experience of having an orgasm in her mind without having her body physically touched. This led to the discovery of her G-spot, which generated much pleasure for both she and Darren.

Profound positive change is a wonderment. When the mind is free to move, the desire felt in a fantasy as it transforms into real experience generates a powerful shift in energy. Like the momentum created by a train locomotive connected to many cars, once it begins moving, it becomes harder to stop. As it reaches a desired cruising speed, there is no doubt it will reach its destination.

Kim learned to go into her mind through hypnosis. She discovered she was capable of experiencing a good healthy sex life with her husband. At the same time she released the emotional and spiritual negative energy from the past. This is what blocked her from the relationship fulfillment she truly wanted. The series of trance experiences allowed her to release the unhealthy messages of guilt and unworthiness. She became free for the positive momentum to build.

The trauma of Trey's death was no longer controlling Kim's sexuality, and the pelvic pain dissolved away. She developed a new energized awareness of herself as a confident woman, embracing life and with a loving passion shared with her husband. The wifely duty of Saturday night sex disappeared over the mountain side.

CHAPTER 6

Childhood Trauma and the Curse

Post-traumatic Stress Disorder (PTSD) as described previously is commonly connected to combat experiences of soldiers during wartime, or to adults responding to emergency situations involving horrific events like 9/11. Obviously, these are not the only situations which can create potential life-threatening fear. PTSD is also frequently discussed as something which occurs relatively soon after the horrific event. This is also not necessarily true. The story of Sean reflects the delayed onset of PTSD by almost three decades, taking him from a child to a 36 year old man. In addition to the usual symptoms including flashbacks, nightmares, irritability, hyper-startle response, and avoidance of related activities, he had to contend with impotency.

Sean's childhood story is presented as graphically detailed as it was described to Dr. Lerman. The intent is to provide an awareness of the severe emotional trauma he experienced, so that there is a common understanding.

Little Sean, as his family affectionately called him, was told by his father to remain in the house with his older sister until his parents returned home with the groceries. This was Belfast, Northern Ireland in July 1972. Sean was eight years old. His sister was 12. Little Sean disobeyed his father and snuck out the back door, climbed the backyard fence and followed his parents, keeping a safe distance out of sight. Seven blocks away, his mother walked into the market and his father went a couple shops further down to a newspaper store.

About 20 minutes later Sean's mother left the market carrying two bags filled with groceries. She yelled for her husband and he came jogging toward her. As they crossed the street a small van sped past them. It sharply turned the corner and the parked car directly in front of his parents exploded into a fiery ball. Sean watched his mother thrown backwards several feet as the groceries flew everywhere. His father dropped to the ground in a heap. The store directly in front of the car burst into flames. Another explosion went off a block away making the ground shake as Sean ran toward his motionless parents lying in the street. People were screaming, some bleeding from cuts. Others were sitting in the gutter moaning in pain. A crowd quickly gathered around his parents and others lying close to the burning car.

Sean fought through the people yelling for his parents. His mother looked like she was asleep. His father was blackened from the blast. His clothes were smoldering and the smell of burning flesh and hair filled Sean's nose as he shook his father trying to revive him. Soon the entire street filled with people. Fire trucks and ambulance sirens wailed. Army trucks carrying soldiers quickly arrived blocking every corner. Seven people died and hundreds were injured by a series of bombs set off by the Irish Republican Army, the IRA, on that day. In the flash of a moment, Sean watched his parents murdered. They were not specifically targeted for attack, simply innocent victims in the wrong place at the wrong time.

The following years of Sean's childhood and young adult years were fairly ordinary. He left Ireland shortly after graduating from college with a degree in business. He was offered a paid internship with a commodities brokerage firm in Chicago owned by a friend of the family. The internship turned into a full-time position and he remained with the company for seven years. He was successful and lived what he labeled "an exciting lifestyle." He also worked hard at creating and maintaining the image of a "playboy," able to use his charming Irish accent and good looks to impress many women. He never considered himself as "the marrying type" and consequently never developed any long-lasting romantic relationships. At the same time he rarely slept alone in his bed.

Sean's world came crashing down when he received word his sister had breast cancer and was gravely ill. They were extremely close, even though she remained in Belfast when he came to America. She very much disapproved of his lifestyle, but remained committed and loving toward him. He hurriedly packed and flew home. On her deathbed she made Sean promise to settle down and have a family to carry on the family name, honoring their parents.

Upon his return to Chicago, Sean began re-defining his life. In order to end the playboy image, he concluded he needed to move. He knew of a contact in Houston looking for a broker to represent his offshore drilling business. He flew down and spent several days in interviews, meetings and getting acquainted with the area. He liked what he experienced and flew back to Chicago with a firm job offer in place. Four weeks later he was on his way to Texas.

Sean quickly acclimated himself to work and began exploring the social life opportunities with the thought of finding a "respectable lass" to pursue a relationship. Being half Jewish by birth, but not raised as a Jew and knowing little about the religion, he had a stereotypic image of Jewish women as 'family oriented.' He believed he would have a good chance of finding potential candidates for a serious relationship by dating several of them.

One of Sean's new co-workers, David, was Jewish. They spent time together talking about life in Houston and women. David invited Sean to his home for dinner to meet his wife, Sharon. She was very active with the Temple and would probably know of any available "respectable lasses." Sure enough there were a few. He planned on joining his new friends at the Temple for the traditional Passover Seder dinner coming up in a couple of weeks.

At the Temple Sean was friendly and engaging. As he helped set up tables and arrange chairs he noticed a woman to the side of the kitchen entrance sitting in a wheelchair. He was instantly attracted to her long wavy red hair. Perhaps it was a positive connection to his childhood.

Sean was not looking at this woman as someone he would want to date, but more of a want to simply connect with and talk. He approached her and extended his hand as he introduced himself. She shook his hand and when she said "Hello" and shared her name, he about melted—Maggie was Irish. She was here visiting her friend, a sorority sister from their years in college together in New York.

Sean and Maggie talked until the Seder started and then well into the night. Each of them was enthralled having someone from their home country to spend time with, even though she was from Dublin and he from Belfast. As small a landmass as Ireland is, the people from Northern Ireland are not typically friendly with those from the south. Fortunately for them, neither of their families identified with the extreme factions and were opposed the history of violence.

Sean and Maggie talked about their careers and experiences coming to America. He was still not looking at her in a romantic way, but felt a connection he had never experienced with a woman before. She had an exciting personality. He felt energized being around her. She seemed to naturally understand him and he caught her finishing his sentences before he could get the words out.

When nine o'clock that evening approached, Maggie told Sean she needed to return to her friend's home. He had no idea they'd spent the past several hours talking. As he rose from his chair, she reached out, took his arm and quietly said, "Kiss me." He leaned forward to politely kiss her forehead. She leaned her head back, placed her hands on either side of his face and met his lips with hers. He felt a jolt of electricity race through his skin. The kiss lasted for several seconds, neither wanting it to end. As they separated she smiled and prepared to leave.

In all his years of being with women, and as suave and "knowing" as Sean prided himself, he had never experienced a moment like that. He called David who listened to Sean ramble on in tangents. David asked how much he had to drink, because he sounded so different. Sean had trouble sleeping that night and called Maggie first thing in the morning. She already committed to spend the day with her friend, but agreed to call him later. They talked and talked until sometime around midnight. Sean was in a trance. He could hardly remember any of what they talked about, but it was a "great discussion."

Sean and Maggie agreed to meet for brunch the next morning at a fitness center. He was supposed to bring his swimsuit, and she was leaving in two days to return to New York. The two messages did not fit together. He chose to only respond to the first. She was waiting for him already in her swimsuit covered by a robe. As they snacked on cheese and fruit, he learned she was a competitive swimmer with the goal of qualifying for the next Paralympics in Australia. It seemed like everything about her was so intriguing and fascinating.

Sean watched as Maggie lowered herself out of the chair into the pool. In her dark gray one-piece suit and swim cap sliding into the water, he imagined she looked like a beautiful seal. Toward the end of their time in the pool, Maggie circled around him underwater coming up to put her hands on his legs and slowly raised them up his body. His arousal was obvious and he was very grateful the pool water came up to his shoulders. She gave him an obvious flirtatious smile, bit him gently on his ear and swam away.

Sean stood motionless in the pool trying to process what was happening. This amazing red headed, green-eyed Irish seal was seducing him! He started after Maggie, but she already reached the ladder and in one smooth motion pulled herself out and into the wheelchair. She removed the swim cap and shook out her hair. He was out of the pool standing in front of her toweling himself. In her chair she was level with his waist and looking directly at his crotch area made the quiet observation, "Little Sean is growing up." He turned beet red. No one had ever assigned a name to his penis before, much less identified it as "Little Sean." He quickly grabbed a handful of towels, wrapped them around his waist and headed for the shower room.

Sean was massively confused. His feelings were all over the place: excited, bewildered, scared, happy, curious and captivated. Thoughts kept racing through his mind. He couldn't focus on anything specific before more thoughts and images flew through his consciousness. What was happening? To David and Sharon it was obvious. They all talked and suggested Sean spend time with Maggie that night to learn what she was experiencing and what direction the two of them wanted to pursue. He called and they agreed to meet at a local Irish tavern.

Maggie was there waiting for Sean at a back corner table. They briefly talked about the quaintness of the tavern and then he took her hand and told her how special she was. He stared into her eyes and told her he didn't want it to end. She agreed. Maggie then told him they needed to know some things about each other. She proceeded to share her story, including the bicycle accident at the age of 12 that caused her paralysis. She severely fractured her pelvic bone and several vertebrae in her lower back.

Maggie refused to use the disabling condition as an excuse for not living her life to its fullest. Swimming allowed her to retain some muscle mass in her legs and nerve functioning in her lower body. She was sexually responsive and the doctors believed she could become pregnant. The only concern would be the need for a Cesarean section delivery.

Sean listened most attentively to Maggie, though not exactly understanding some of the medical information. She wanted to know more about his childhood and family. He brushed this aside beyond sharing the factual material of his parents' death, playing soccer, close relationship with his sister and staying in the home of his aunt until going off to the university.

That night, Maggie's last in Houston before returning to her home in New York, they returned to Sean's apartment and made love. It was passionate and tender. In bed, her agility and body control amazed him. Their climaxes were far beyond what either previously experienced. In the morning they said goodbye with the promise to talk after she arrived home.

For the next three months Sean and Maggie talked on the phone every night. They became Instant Messengers over the Internet. He had two weeks of vacation so they planned for him to spend the time with her in New York. He was familiar with New York from several business trips before and enjoyed the visits, but they were nothing compared to the excitement of exploring the city with Maggie.

Sean and Maggie would not see each other again until the end of the fall semester, four months away. The long distance relationship was extremely taxing for both of them. When mid-December finally arrived he was so antsy, David would ask every morning at work if he had taken his "chill pill" yet. With her arrival he lightened up. They were so much in love and wanted to maximize every moment, knowing how precious their time together meant. On New Year's Eve he asked her to marry him and gave her a ring. She was thrilled and overwhelmed. Two days later they said goodbye again, planning on being together in New York for the spring break.

In the middle of training and preparation for a Paralympics-qualifying swim meet, Maggie became sick and was hospitalized with a blood disorder and severe anemia. Sean rushed to New York. The sight of her in the hospital bed frightened him. The grayish skin tone caused a flashback to seeing his sister just before her death. Even Maggie's usual electrifying smile was not right. Her emerald green eyes were not glistening. Despite hearing all the assurances from her and the liver doctor, about the predicted full recovery, he felt like he was collapsing inside.

Sean had already lost the three most important people in his life, and the fear of losing Maggie became overwhelming. In his state of fear he started racking his brain, looking for any possible understanding. He wondered if perhaps someone put a curse on him while he was a boy. Cursing is a fairly common aspect of Irish mythology, and he remembered some of the old people talking about how their lives were cursed. Of course, he thought it was nonsense, but in this moment of fear, all things seemed possible.

Sean became withdrawn and reclusive. His work effort dropped off. The evening talks with Maggie felt conflicted and ended far sooner than in the past. The strain on the relationship intensified. He began having nightmares of growing up in Belfast. There were monsters threatening to eat people and stealing children away from their homes. The dreams were in black and white and all the people had gray skin and sad faces. Evil leprechauns shouted vile curses at pregnant women.

Sean met with his physician, who assured him he was simply going through a "tough time" because of the separation from Maggie. He felt somewhat better and left the doctor's office headed to a pharmacy with prescriptions for sleeping pills and depression. He slept through the night for the first time in quite a while with no bad dreams. He was still lethargic, but expected the anti-depressant medication would take several days to build up in his system, as his physician explained. So he patiently waited for the relief to come. It was marginal, at best. Maggie decided to visit him as soon as her school semester ended.

Sean and Maggie were happy to see each other, but something was very wrong. There was no excitement and no passion. They talked about wanting to re-connect, but it was not the same as before. She started seeing a psychotherapist to help her cope with the frustrating effects of her illness and disappointment of missing the Paralympics. She shared her belief that Sean also needed therapy. He initially resisted the idea because he had no understanding of it. By the end of the evening Sean agreed to see someone.

As Sean and Maggie were greeted in Dr. Lerman's waiting room, Maggie gave Sean a reassuring nod sending him on his way. He was somewhat uncomfortable, acknowledging he had no idea of what to expect. In the session they talked about work and the difficulties keeping a long distance relationship fresh. As Sean went back reviewing the early history of the relationship, his mood perked up. He had no problem explaining his excitement as the infatuation ignited. The stress of the current relationship status was obvious. However, there was something very unsettled and troubling under the surface from how Sean talked about the problems with Maggie.

Sean listened to the options of traditional cognitive therapy versus hypnotherapy. He jokingly asked if hypnosis could remove curses and hexes, then chose to keep the therapy in the conscious field. We would come back to his believed curse much later, when he was ready. During the initial course of therapy he learned effective stress management strategies. His work performance re-energized. He was getting to bed earlier and sleeping through the night. His daily life became far less stressful.

The last couple days of Maggie's visit were pleasant and caring, but not particularly passionate. During their last two sexual experiences Sean's potency level was so restricted he had difficulty becoming aroused and lost his erection without climax. He dismissed these episodes as just feeling tired and she accepted it because they were feeling closer. It bothered him a great deal. He had never encountered erectile difficulty before, but because he was feeling better on the surface, he chose to ignore the problem.

Sean stated he had completed what he needed concerning his stress and wanted to stop therapy. He agreed there were still conflict areas, and once he had clearer understanding of his relationship, he would get back in contact to schedule his next appointment. On September 14, 2001, three days following 9/11, he called to schedule an emergency appointment. He was a nervous wreck. There was no communication from Maggie for the three previous days. Even though he knew the school she taught at and her apartment were not close to the lower end of Manhattan, the fear of the moment overwhelmed him.

This time Sean openly talked about "The Curse." It was the one he imposed on himself for disobeying his father the day his parents died. He cursed himself to never receive love again. His unconscious mind constructed a wall to protect him from the hurt of losing someone he loved. Each time he saw the rubble of the World Trade Center and the gray ashen people, flashbacks of losing his parents came to the forefront of his mind.

Sean startled awake from a terrifying dream, smelling the burnt hair and skin of his father. The sound of the explosions kept ringing in his ears. Almost like a slow motion replay, he saw his mother falling backwards and the groceries flying away from her. All of his senses were in a heightened state of arousal and he could not shut it off. He feared losing his mind, or worse, going back in time to re-live those horrifying moments over and over again. It was time for Sean to confront and release his curse.

All clients provide suggestions or cues for the therapist to engage the hypnosis process. Sometimes it is the words used to describe an event, or the importance of an event. Sometimes it is a specific or unique quality. Irish heritage is rich in mythology involving stories of slaying dragons and evil entities, along with unicorns and mermaids. There are plenty of potential metaphors available to draw from. The key identifiers would involve those on which Sean placed a high value. He provided many powerful symbols in reporting his history and sharing the nightmares.

The goal of utilizing the symbols was to reframe Sean's childhood trauma away from the guilt reaction attributed to not obeying his father. Within the mythology stories bad things happen to innocent people. Witches caste evil curses, leprechauns steal children, and dragon burn down village homes. Sean would find himself taking on the hero qualities of the valiant young warrior. Unconsciously, he knew he could not undo his parents' deaths; however, he could restore peace of mind and allow himself to release the emotional horror reaction as being his fault.

Several stories followed in which the hero from long ago engaged in battles with an evil witch, a mean spirited leprechaun, and a fire-breathing dragon. With each battle Sean would drive out the bad influences. One story would start and become embedded into another story. Unconsciously, he processed the meaning as his imagination integrated the metaphors into a level of intuitive understanding.

Sean's unconscious mind began identifying solutions for resolving the emotional power of the trauma with minimal coaching. His imagination focused on the outcomes of the stories, applying them to his life experiences. As he conquered the evil forces, he began releasing the negative emotional bond of the trauma. Positive healing energy allowed Sean to transpose from a victim to a hero, no longer shackled to self-imposed guilt.

Sean could now to focus his attention on Maggie and the loss of sexual desire and performance. Although displays of affection improved during her last visit, there was no want for sex. He felt selfish talking about his sex drive problem while Maggie dealt with the aftermath of the tragedy in New York. At that particular time, there was no value pursuing the sexual issue. He wanted to be with her and keep her safe, knowing very well there was nothing he could do to protect her from another terrorist attack.

Sean received counseling assistance to pull together an action plan for lowering his stress, similar to the cognitive therapy when he first started seeing Dr. Lerman. He knew he would need Maggie's input to create a plan for being with her. He understood his immediate need was to reach out to Maggie in love, not fear. She called him that night and they talked.

Sean and Maggie worked out a plan for them to be together in the near future on a more permanent basis. Once the safety issue was resolved, Sean was able to address his sexual dysfunction. While in trance he learned how to remain in the present and respond only to his sensory cues of sight, touch, sound, smell and taste. All conscious thought was replaced by his unconscious awareness of how his biology naturally worked, free from thinking. After the third session, Sean developed a quick self-hypnosis program in his mind that he would practice before engaging in sexual activity with Maggie.

Follow up phone calls reflected Sean and Maggie's continued progress and growth together. They married that summer. Several months later Maggie became pregnant. She gave birth to a healthy son, named Samuel, after Sean's father. Three years later their daughter Heather was born, named in memory of Maggie's mother. Sean fulfilled the promise to his sister. The curse was ancient history. He was loved and he embraced it.

Sean learned a great deal about himself through the hypnotherapy process. He had no conscious awareness of the impact his past had on his present life. He was only able to focus on the surface level of stress. He didn't realize that there was a connection between the childhood trauma, his sister's death, and the feared loss of Maggie.

Even though he joked about the possibility of being cursed before seriously dismissing it, he knew at the unconscious level that something in him was significantly interfering with his relationship. Sean's discovery of his unconscious mind enabled him to shift from the immediate panic about Maggie, to the release of the negative images and messages about his worthiness to receive love.

CHAPTER 7

Permanent Weight Control

Obsession. This is the most dominant word describing America's attitude toward weight loss. There is a never-ending supply of weight loss programs with their 'before and after' pictures and claims of success filling television and radio ad space. If anything related to weight can be measured, there is a need to know it and buy something to reduce it or enhance it. Numbers take on magical importance. The obsession demands that people 'count carbs,' follow cholesterol 'ranges,' weigh themselves daily, and purchase supplements based on parts per million of vitamin content; but how many apples a day *really* keeps the doctor away?

Catch-phrases about nutrition don't stop there. 'Red wine is good for your heart,' but, 'alcohol is bad for your liver.' 'Coffee will wake you up,' but, 'caffeine crashes give you the jitters.' Parents want their children healthy and happy, and yet children's connection between food and happiness centers on refined sugar, saturated- and trans-fats, and complex carbs. The bombardment of diet-related messages by media fuels the obsession, and the contradictory messages create confusion. How can good parents deny 'happy' meals to their children?

People spend money on all kinds of weight loss remedies wanting to believe that they can make it work. Most lose some weight initially, but once the excitement wears off, people's previous emotional states like boredom, self-doubt, unresolved anger, and discontent resurface, and the weight loss stops. Sometimes, if the weight loss is too rapid, the mind will slow the body's metabolism to prevent more weight loss, because it generates a physical reaction as if starvation is happening. After a period of no progress, people feel discouraged and as the previous negative emotions build, the old eating habits return, along with weight gain.

The critical issue with weight control is that it has nothing to do with 'loss.' The word itself implies a negative experience. When we lose something, we usually make a concerted effort to 'find it!' When it comes to pounds and inches, we can almost always find what we have lost. In fact, most overweight people are masters of finding what they've lost. One of Dr. Lerman's clients calculated he had lost more than 1,000 pounds in his 30-year pursuit of weight loss.

The commitment to controlling weight is not simply a conscious goal of will power or New Year's resolution. It is part of the path to permanently achieving good health. Sustaining the commitment requires the active participation of the unconscious mind to involve intuitive knowledge, imagination, creativity, altered feeling states, and biological changes. The stories of Angie and Terry are consistent with thousands of adults who achieve permanent results utilizing hypnosis to incorporate the conscious and unconscious mind.

Angie

Angie requested hypnotherapy to help her control her weight. During each of her three pregnancies she gained 45-50 pounds. Unfortunately, she only lost 30 pounds after the first, 20 after the second and little to none after the third. She was 100 pounds heavier than what she weighed on her wedding day.

Despite numerous efforts of sustained dieting and workout routines, several physician assisted medication regimens and participation in store-front weight loss programs, nothing worked over time. Typically, Angie would drop 20-30 pounds at the start of each new effort, eventually hit a plateau and then gradually re-gain all the weight back. She registered with a bariatric surgery program, thinking that was the last resort. Her insurance company refused to consider paying any part of it, until she participated in a medically supervised weight reduction program for one full year.

The thought of surgery scared the heck out of Angie, but she was reaching a point of desperation typical of many middle-aged obese adults. The combined effect of aching joints, little physical stamina, mental fatigue, social rejection, low self-esteem, ongoing frustration, high blood pressure, hypoglycemia and diabetes became overwhelming. She believed she could handle the surgery. However, waiting a whole year while taking another medication, more lab work, and having to see a doctor once a month seemed so illogical. She had already done this routine several times.

Angie's husband, Tom, heard a work colleague talk about his success losing a great deal of weight several years ago. He worked with a clinical hypnotist. Tom went on the Internet and did some research. He learned about the mind/body connection and how healthy results are obtained without medication and rigid diet plans. He then raised the option with her.

Since Angie was still eleven months away from surgery, assuming the insurance company would approve it then, she figured she might as well see if it could help. As an actuarial accountant, she quickly determined the cost would be less expensive than the continued physician visits, lab fees, medications and co-payment the insurance company would require after she paid the annual deductible—and that didn't include her out-of-pocket cost for the actual surgery.

Effective hypnotherapy is not a 'one size fits all' scripted process. There are several different approaches and techniques available. During the "pre-talk" when the client and clinician initially discuss the client's desired result, there are many facets for the clinician to explore to determine a specific approach. Understanding clients' spoken and unspoken messages, how easily they access their imagination and the emotional inner-connection to eating are critical parts.

For Angie, overeating was the result of long-standing emotional stress. The behavior was intended to soothe sadness, worry, fear, anger, resentment, rejection and abandonment. It was also used to insulate from memories of deeply hurtful events. Some people overeat only in the evenings after work, or once the children are put to bed, as a reaction to boredom or loneliness. Some people eat continuously throughout the day, in order to feel nurtured due to the absence of positive loving relationships. Some people eat continuously over weekends and on holidays to mask grief from a lost or ended relationship. Some people overeat to soothe shame. Interspersed with these factors are habitual patterns of poor food choices, minimal or inaccurate dietary knowledge, exercise avoidance, passive-aggression toward self and others, along with a myriad of self-justifying, irrational self-talk messages.

During the initial session Angie identified her usual eating habits and many emotional triggers. She rarely ate breakfast at home, always rushing to get the children up, off to school and on her way to work. Tom left the house an hour before the rest of the family got up to beat the morning rush hour traffic. Every morning she would hit the drive-thru coffee shop to get "energized." At work, there were donuts and sometimes bagels and cream cheese awaiting her. This would "sustain" her until the mid-morning break, which was pretty much a repeat of breakfast. Lunch was her only nutritious meal of the day.

Dinner time was hectic because one child had dance class and Girl Scout meetings, another was in T-ball or soccer and the third was in an after-school reading development program. The dinner meal was either fast food take out or something from the freezer section of the grocery store. Weekends were similarly hectic with shopping, house cleaning, laundry, yard work, and hopefully a date night with her husband. Mealtime preparation rarely existed except for the Sunday dinners involving her parents or in-laws.

Angie did not give herself permission to relax. Numbing out in the evenings watching TV, replying to Facebook posts from friends and relatives, snacking on high-carb foods and drinking a large glass of wine was not relaxation. This became the first clinical priority. It took Angie almost 30 minutes listening to Dr. Lerman's relaxation suggestions before she allowed herself to relax. As she experienced her body releasing tension, her mind struggled to release the ever present negative racing thoughts.

The trance messages given to Angie encouraged her to make sure everything was done and in its place. The Biblical story of Noah was introduced as a metaphor. She imagined that all the hard work to build the ark and round up the animals was done. The animals were safely on board and the soft sound of rain was hitting the roof of the boat. It was okay for her to let go now. Unfortunately, only a few minutes later her conscious mind intruded into the peacefulness. It questioned what to do should the animals not get along, how the stalls would be cleaned, and how the larger animals would get exercise. We do learn from our clients!

These pragmatic, logical messages were typical of what prevented Angie from relaxing and focusing on her health. They represented two deeply engrained beliefs. The first was she always had to be doing something productive, so there was no time for relaxation. The second belief was that her value as a human being was only derived from what she did for others. There was no value for self-care or self-love. That was shameful and selfish. The session went far beyond the allotted time. However, the strategy for reaching an effective result was now understood. At the end of the session, Angie received a relaxation CD with the instruction to listen to it every night.

To begin the next session Angie reported not feeling any better. She questioned whether she was a good candidate for hypnosis. This is a common reaction for people locked into a negative belief system of not deserving good things for themselves. Angie stated she only listened to the CD the evening following the session, claiming to forget to set up the CD player after that. Bypassing anymore of her negative "self-less" report, Dr. Lerman intentionally focused only on the first night. She smiled as she talked about sleeping soundly for eight hours. When the alarm clock went off, she awoke feeling refreshed and full of energy. She applied the energy in the kitchen, and made scrambled eggs and cut up fresh fruit for her children. She ate breakfast with them for the first time in a very long time.

For the second session Angie received a slightly different message: "Wouldn't it be interesting, if the good feeling you have knowing your husband is getting a good night's rest, became an even better good feeling knowing you are having a good night's rest?" She settled into the trance and received another embedded message: "As you go deeper into the trance, you might experience seeing your husband smiling in a most approving way, and at some point in the near future, perhaps within 30 seconds or maybe 20 seconds, your smiling face can be right next to his." In about 30 seconds Angie smiled and relaxed very deeply into hypnosis.

The trance suggestion did not specifically focus on releasing the negative messages. The intention of the suggestions was to emphasize more positive feelings and transfer self-care into Angie's beliefs. While scheduling her next appointment, she promised to listen to the CD every night when going to bed.

When Angie arrived for her next visit she looked very calm and reported sleeping better and feeling more energized. Taking her into a working trance now became an easy task and one she positively anticipated. Multiple stories involving metaphors of letting go ensued, each intended to loosen her negative beliefs. Also embedded within the stories, were messages of self-care, self-nurturing and self-love. One specific story she found especially motivating involved a theme of relaxing by water. The combined effect of visualizing herself around a waterfall and drinking cool spring water was a powerful suggestion for her to remain calm and relaxed. It also reinforced the nutritional need to drink plenty of water. Obese people typically do not drink enough water. They commonly misinterpret the message for thirst as one for hunger and default to eating.

In addition to the metaphor lined stories, Angie received post-hypnotic suggestions to recognize when she felt valued preparing home cooked meals, and satisfied eating smaller portions of healthy foods. There were also suggestions that she would always sit down before eating, chew her food slowly and enjoy the taste of each bite.

Within four weeks the family was eating home cooked breakfasts and dinners several times a week. Angie discovered the crock pot that had been gathering dust in the pantry for the previous 12 years was really a tremendous aid. She prepared large dinners on Sunday and by freezing the leftovers had a second meal for later in the week. Tom often smoked and grilled meat and fish on Saturdays. He started filling the smoker with food. After enjoying the meal, the extras were frozen. It took little time to heat up and serve with store prepared bags of salad or microwavable vegetables on weekdays.

Angie was shedding the excess pounds and inches and she became happier and healthier. She also walked the outside perimeter of her son's baseball field or soccer field while he practiced, rather than sitting in the vehicle texting or in the bleachers talking with the other moms. Eventually, three of the moms joined her in the walks and they became good friends. The true test for Angie was not the weight loss, but her acceptance of becoming healthier over time. Within 11 months she successfully said good bye to 78 pounds, and completed her first of many 10K walks to support various charitable health awareness causes. Two years following her initial hypnosis session, her weight leveled off at 90 pounds less than when she started. It did not fluctuate more than a couple pounds from one week to the next.

The key to Angie's weight control success was the shift in her focus away from the concept of dieting which is a message of deprivation and self-denial. Instead, the primary messages she internalized and experienced related to valuing herself, while releasing the negative beliefs. She empowered her mind and body to become healthy. As Angie embraced the awareness of freedom from negative beliefs, she became the person she wanted to be. She still took care of her family, and now she cared about herself as well. She was in full control and loved her life.

Terry

The need to be in control for an athlete is a message taught very early in training. The competitive spirit demands mental conditioning, and rejects loss as an acceptable outcome. Helping a former athlete gain control over a weight problem was not about loss. It was designed to create a victory.

Terry arrived at Dr. Lerman's office six months after his company's purchasing department became a casualty of 'down-sizing.' The owners sold the business to another company. Suddenly, instead of having a satisfying career and secure job, he had no income. A family used to a comfortable lifestyle had with no means to support it. The shocking awareness of his devalued work experience seriously damaged his ego. Although his wife and children remained supportive, and willingly let go of many of the conveniences they grew to take for granted, it ate at him every day. The chronic stress affected him in ways he did not know.

As a 43 year old man, Terry was competing against younger candidates for positions he supervised the past 12 years. He strongly believed the extra 60 pounds of weight he carried was a serious distraction to potential employers.

Although Terry presented a positive attitude about his abilities and had a long history of professional accomplishments, his feelings of inadequacy in not providing for the family were seriously draining his daily efforts. His head hunter referred him for hypnotherapy to address the weight issue and restore his self-esteem and confidence.

Terry was a large man even without the extra weight. He was an amateur wrestler throughout high school and college, winning many medals and competitions. He prided himself on staying in good shape well into his late 30s. He loved playing racquetball and handball with the same competitive desire to win. He also repeatedly crashed into the walls and dove onto the hard floors. He suffered torn ligaments in both a shoulder and a knee. They required surgery and prolonged physical inactivity. His solid muscle structure began turning to fat. At the same time his appetite remained the same and the weight gain started.

When Terry arrived for the initial appointment, his face and neck areas were beet red, and he complained about feeling exhausted. The elevators in the office building were out of order, and he climbed the single flight of stairs to the second floor office. His last physical exam was more than a year past, and much had changed in his life since then. Terry was asked several health-related questions that indicated he sometimes had difficulty breathing, and he often felt his heart pounding from engaging in light physical activity. There were other responses further suggesting a possible heart problem.

Terry followed suggestions to breathe deeper and slower to increase the flow of oxygen throughout his body, and allow him to relax. He responded well to a guided imagery technique placing him on a beautiful beach, and completely released all the pressure in his mind and body. He appeared significantly calmer. The redness disappeared and he reported feeling better, free from the racing sensation he had a few minutes earlier. His breathing was easy and slow.

Terry signed a release of information allowing Dr. Lerman to speak with his physician, and a call was immediately made to the physician's office. Once the symptoms were conveyed to the doctor's nurse, she quickly got the physician on the phone. He spoke with Terry and scheduled to see him first thing the next morning. The physician felt there was no need for emergency hospital care, but made sure Terry had his after-hours phone number just in case.

At 7:45 the next morning Terry was at his physician's office. His blood pressure was high, but no other symptoms indicated a need for critical care or continuous monitoring. He left with a prescription to bring down the blood pressure and a referral for hypnotherapy. At the next session Terry described his high school and college wrestling experiences as the best times of his life. He loved the conditioning program, the competition, and learning to master the techniques of balancing strength and finesse. This would become the basis of several metaphors related to him regaining the balance in his life.

Amateur wrestling is a highly competitive sport, very much different than the staged 'professional' events reflected in Wrestle Mania and pay-per-view television broadcasts. These young athletes follow practice and conditioning programs similar to the training of high school and collegiate football players. The most obvious difference is that the wrestlers compete individually and are matched to opponents of the same weight. The skills and techniques are of equal importance to strength, speed and stamina. Having the ability to anticipate an opponent's move provides a distinct advantage for body positioning, leverage and control.

While in trance Terry imagined himself in a match. He utilized all his skills and most importantly, accurately anticipated his opponent's moves. The anticipation resulted from the activation of his intuitive knowledge and unconsciously created the balance he needed. He identified a wrist sweatband as an anchoring reminder to maintain his mind in a centered and balanced state.

Within three sessions the weight reduction started, and Terry felt better with more confidence and control. On his way to a job interview, he intentionally wore the sweatband all the way to the office and removed it as he walked through the interviewer's door. The interview went very well, however, he was not offered that specific job. The company was in the process of opening a new office and he would be brought in to interview with the new manager. He took the news as a positive challenge and began a mental and physical conditioning program. Coming in for a follow up session, he focused on excelling in presenting himself as confident. He created a powerful image of participating in the Olympics and winning the gold medal.

During the eight week period of time involving the four sessions, Terry lost 25 pounds. The internal balance and confidence became powerful. He received the job offer and interestingly turned it down. He opted to join one of his former co-workers in a consulting business, so he could become his own boss. The rest of the weight came off within the next four months and he returned to a modified racquetball program.

Terry overcame adversity through mental change. It reflected the kind of strength the unconscious mind is capable of exerting when it is allowed to naturally work. His successful experiences as an athlete were part of his past experience. In his unconscious mind he possessed knowledge of the characteristics and qualities necessary to solve his present situation. He knew he could be self-reliant and self-dependent.

As Terry experienced himself in trance, he re-discovered his mental strengths and re-learned to trust his intuition. As he embraced the positive images and feelings about himself, he released the negative feelings of doubt and guilt, and lack of self-worth. The use of the sweatband reminded him of who he was and what he was capable of achieving. He allowed the creativity and imagination in his unconscious mind to find the best solutions.

The post-hypnotic suggestions about healthy eating and portion control became natural and easily accepted. There was no doubt in Terry's mind he was ready to experience success. He learned to welcome change and won a life-altering victory.

CHAPTER 8

Driven to Dysfunction

Why does life seem so hard to balance? Just when one part is running well, another part is in crisis. Even when all of the rules for achieving success are followed, failure can still happen. Sacrifices are made with the intention of making the future better. However, without understanding the value of what is sacrificed, there may be nothing left to 'make better' in the future. Doug's story is an unfortunately common one. He succeeded in building an executive career, but at the expense of both his marriage and his family.

Doug was a bright, good looking man in his 40's who rapidly climbed the corporate ladder. He was seemingly a perfect example of the modern success story. When Doug first met his future wife, Vickie, she was a school teacher. After they became engaged, she agreed to give up her career, and direct her attention toward supporting him and raising their future children. They had two beautiful daughters and lived in a suburban dream house with an envious lifestyle. Despite the glistening surface, there was a disaster waiting to happen.

Doug provided well for his wife and children, and they enjoyed their improving lifestyle. However, he had no regard for the value of his time or the importance of marriage and family. His frequent absences from home and missing the children's important activities were defended as regretful, but necessary;

always followed by the promise that someday it would all be worth it.

As Doug obsessed over building an impressive career, he became more and more oblivious to the deteriorating quality of his home life. He was more married to his job than to Vickie, and more pre-occupied by his work than his children's needs for a father. Frequent pleadings for more of Doug's attention turned ugly. It became a constant stream of nagging, blaming, and ridicule. The last eight years of his 12-year marriage mutated into a nightmare.

Doug's defensiveness at home included criticisms about Vickie's ingratitude and inability to understand that he was working hard to provide a better life for their family. In turn, she accused him of having affairs as well as an addiction to pornography, along with several other possibilities her sister and mid-day television programs suggested. These destructive exchanges went on for years. Over time, he became bewildered, confused and resentful.

Not surprisingly, Doug's and Vickie's sex life followed the downward trajectory of their marriage. It went from a mutually satisfying, passionate, exciting and bonding experience, to an occasional, unenthusiastic 'let's do it and get it over with,' concession. In the beginning of the marriage, several times a year Doug arranged for Vickie to accompany him to out-of-town business meetings. It helped re-ignite their passion. As time conflicts with their children's activities became more common, she stopped going with him. Their passion vanished. Even the obligatory sexual encounters disappeared and there was no intimacy of any kind.

Vickie initiated marriage counseling on two occasions. Although Doug readily agreed to attend, work demands were a greater priority. In a moment of exasperation, he exclaimed he could not be expected to keep scheduled appointments—a message he would never consider making at work. As a couple they were unable to participate in, and benefit from professional help. This, paired with the absence of closeness and even basic kindness, destroyed any hope of saving their marriage.

Angry verbal attacks continued well after the divorce. There was no truth to Vickie's claims of Doug's infidelity or addiction to pornography, but fear and resentful anger rarely lend themselves to facts or sound reasoning. Neither one of them would let go or stop blaming the other. The children begged their mother to let them live with their grandparents, even after the divorce, so they could get away from the anger and yelling. Doug and Vickie were spiraling into deepening mud, and unable to move on with their respective lives.

Doug initially found dating completely unsatisfying, especially with a non-existent sex drive. Three years after the divorce, he began seeing Sharon, a minister's widow. Doug very much enjoyed her supportive and unassuming demeanor, but remained unable to refrain from belligerent remarks about Vickie. As they spent more time together, Sharon wanted to advance their relationship. She suggested that he needed help forgiving his ex-wife, so they could move forward as a couple. He agreed, but took no action. His resentful comments returned a few weeks later and caused so much discomfort for Sharon, that she repeated the same suggestion again with an even greater sense of urgency.

While Doug's pattern of avoidance continued, Sharon learned about a workshop offered by a neighboring church. It focused on the theme of forgiveness after marriages end. Doug's job was temporarily less demanding. Since he wasn't working Sunday evenings planning for the coming week, and football season was over, his common excuses didn't work. After attending all four parts of the program, Doug claimed he felt freed from harboring any more ill-will toward Vickie.

Doug very much wanted to please Sharon, but he had not completely released his negative energy. The anger was burrowed deep inside his unconscious mind and no amount of conscious will power was going to let it go. The only effect Doug's participation in the workshop had on his behavior was a reduction in the number of angry outbursts he made about Vickie. Finding forgiveness was only superficial.

Several months into the relationship, Sharon sought to take matters into her own hands. During an evening of much wine and heated passion, she seduced him and they attempted intercourse. Doug lost his erection within a few minutes. Sharon's feelings were hurt, but she remained supportive. He felt embarrassed and tremendously inadequate.

Sharon and Doug believed his erectile problem was a fluke and attributed it to fatigue and perhaps, too much wine. They tried once more, and again experienced the same result.

After a couple more unsuccessful attempts, Doug became overwhelmed with self-doubt and worry. He feared that he'd never be able to perform. They prayed about it and consulted the church pastor. The pastor listened attentively, prayed with them, and referred Doug to a physician specializing in internal medicine. The physician offered a trial sample of male enhancement pills with instructions for their use.

Doug's initial reaction to the medication was positive. He sustained an erection through climax during intercourse with Sharon. Unfortunately, he developed two negative side-effects as time went on. First, he had headaches each time he took the medication. Second, his erections became less and less potent. The physician responded by changing the prescription, but the results were even more negative. The headaches became more intense, and his blood pressure escalated to an unsafe level. In order to increase blood flow to his penis, the heart was pumping too fast.

Doug's physician prescribed Xanax, an anti-anxiety medication, also known by its generic name alprazolam, to offset the negative side-effects of the enhancement pills. Continual usage of Xanax can cause chemical addiction. Doug entangled himself in a dangerous situation by taking medication cocktails in order to perform sexually. He also identified a noticeable decrease in mental sharpness at work, as a side-effect of the added medication.

Rationally, Doug concluded that there had to be a better alternative than dependency on medications. For several months, he had heard a radio spot promoting hypnosis for relationship issues, but dismissed it as nonsense. That was before the onset of his erectile dysfunction and difficulties with medication side-effects. He called Dr. Lerman's office to schedule an initial appointment for a 'relationship problem.'

At the start of the session it was unclear why Doug had come. 'Relationship problem' is a rather broad and non-specific topic. Most often it is the female partner who calls to schedule the first session. From Dr. Lerman's experience, when men call to work on a relationship problem, it is typically because they have been served with divorce papers and are very confused, they've found out their partner has had an affair, their partner is already seeing a therapist and the man decides he needs one also, the couple is gay, or there is a sexual dysfunction problem. About half the male callers will clearly state they have an erectile or sexual problem.

Doug's initial presentation at the office was one of arrogance and false pride—something more belonging to a stereotypic boardroom meeting of junior executives trying to impress the company CEO. As much as he wanted the help, his mind was determined to protect his ego. Dr. Lerman casually suggested he might try taking two deep breaths and as he slowly let the air out the second time, to think about the 10 words or less he could use to explain why he was there. Following a momentary stare of confusion, Doug took the deep breaths and then very slowly muttered, "I've have ED."

Confession is not only good for the soul. It does wonders for clarifying the client's need. It also allows the therapist to begin establishing the trust that would enable Doug to provide all the rich, though painful background history. From this information a clinical plan emerged for the hypnotic trance to become most effective in encouraging the internal changes to happen.

During the session, it was determined that Doug's erectile problem was perpetuated by several issues related to stress and guilt. All of them could be resolved by engaging his unconscious mind. Due to Doug's exceptionally analytical nature, he over-relied on logical thinking. However, this kind of analysis applied to sexuality only created more stress because biological functioning does not improve with increased thinking.

At the start of the second session, Doug was encouraged to focus all of his mental energy on the desired results. He was coached to imagine what it would be like once his virility and sexual confidence were fully restored. He listened as he was guided through a maze of increasing confusion. In the process of trying to keep up with the distorted logic, he released the need to rationally understand and allowed his conscious mind to rest. His unconscious mind created a very safe internal place, as he released all physical and mental tension.

Doug imagined an internal storehouse becoming the center for confidence, positive energy, sexual strength, and fulfillment. It was his special treasure house. He would always know this place existed within him. In order to find it, Dr. Lerman presented a metaphor enhanced story during trance. Doug fought and hacked his way through a jungle creating a path to his personal treasure house. He learned a self-hypnosis technique that allowed him to continue working on his path in between sessions.

The metaphor drew an illusion between the conflicts, false accusations, and negativity in Doug's life, with common aspects of a scary jungle. These personal problems and other obstacles became poisonous vines, bat-infested trees, thorny shrubs, and huge nasty spider webs. In order for Doug to reach his treasure house, he had to confront the conflicts, resolve the problems, and clear the obstacles of his Amazon.

The most significant matter for Doug to address concerned his marriage to Vicky. Before he could forgive his ex-wife, he had to recognize and take responsibility for his part in the events that lead to their divorce. He finally understood the impact his tunnel vision had on their relationship. Once the emotional reality of his actions 'hit home,' he opened up to exploring for further insight.

Doug found three remaining obstacles. First, he acknowledged and released the faulty and rigid expectations he placed on himself. Second, he understood that the defeating limitations he experienced directly resulted from his narrow definition of success. Third, he gained awareness as to how willingly he accepted the excessive expectations others imposed on him at work. The resolutions to these issues enabled him to clear a pathway, creating his chosen direction in life.

Doug replaced the false bravado with a more humble, compassionate presentation. He remained just as determined to succeed, but his depth and range of view greatly expanded. His analytic mind improved as he was able to absorb more intuitive information, and discovered the relief of not needing to know all the answers.

Once Doug allowed his shifting mind to reorganize and reprioritize, the sexual problem easily became solvable. He realized he couldn't sustain an erection by thinking about it, any more than he could prevent losing it. Then he understood that as soon as he started thinking about sex, he created a negative expectation to fail, which he mastered. While in trance he accessed the creative part of his unconscious mind and found the solution—he could focus only on the immediate experience of how his body was reacting and allow the passion to naturally build. He didn't need to know why worked, if he was getting what he wanted.

The final step in Doug's healing process was for him to learn self-hypnosis. He could then continue to access the inner solutions and reinforce all the new learning he was incorporating into his life. In the process he found forgiveness for Vickie and began re-building healthy, loving relationships with his daughters. The healing went far beyond the original 'relationship problem,' which is often the case when hypnosis is allowed to access the unconscious mind.

Doug reported no further sexual problems. He and Sharon married shortly thereafter and established a great sex life. He is presently the vice president of sales and marketing for a Fortune 500 company and thoroughly enjoys his life. Doug embraced a healthy decision when he made balancing life's roles a priority. This balance sustains the natural flow of energy between the mind and body. Catering to imposed obligations disrupts the mind/body connection and creates dysfunction.

Sexual desire and performance are natural functions of the mind. When conflicting messages override the mind's stability, the solution is not found in pills. The goal is to understand and re-establish the flow of energy. On a limited basis, medication can be effective for men who actually need to increase blood flow to the penis—those typically over the age of 60, or those diagnosed with blood pressure problems. However, sexual performance is more than simply getting hard and sustaining an erection.

A man's sexual strength is rooted in his unconscious mind. Hypnosis is an extremely effective tool for reaching this place and encouraging positive changes to happen as negative energy and messages are released. When sex is great, men and women are in balanced trance states, experiencing their own treasure house.

CHAPTER 9

Look Like a Model

The idea of teenagers and young adults starving themselves is frightening, and beyond logical understanding. An obsession with body image can be devastating. Anorexia Nervosa involves an extreme mental and behavioral reaction to an intense fear of being fat. The mind becomes so stressed that normal perceptions of sight, smell, and taste are distorted into false illusions. Eating one piece of lettuce, or a single cherry tomato is believed to be a filling salad. Eating a single peanut is interpreted as if it were a whole peanut butter sandwich.

The mindset can last well into young adulthood, and has the potential to prompt fatal behaviors. There is no rational argument that can convince a person with anorexia to see what is actually happening. When highly vulnerable, self-conscious children and adolescents internalize the messages and images preoccupied with thinness, the fear of being fat becomes overwhelmingly powerful.

Turn on the television. Look through popular magazines. Check out the models prancing their way across the screen or posing on the pages spread before you. What they have in common is that they are almost painfully thin. They make fortunes modeling and often springboard from the runway into the fashion world to create their own design labels. Many achieve 'A-List' stardom and marry famous athletes and other celebrities. These fashion models lead by example for millions of suggestible pre-adolescents and teens from both genders. What young person today doesn't dream of achieving this kind of fame and wealth?!

The 'thin is beautiful' message, from the 1960's is even more exaggerated in present times with the absence of parental involvement and guidance. Many parents accept unreasonable working demands in efforts to maintain a more comfortable lifestyle for their children. Their struggles are further complicated by constant worries over finances, and conflicted relationships with significant others. The picture these parents model for their children is one of uncertainty and constant chaos. As the stress persists, their children internalize the message that it is okay, and even normal, to be out of control. Sustaining this rat race at the expense of regular discussions about values, minimal quality time, and consistent limit setting, encourages young people to rely more on peers and media for information and standards of appearance.

Youngsters caught between the attraction to the fashion model glamour, and the parent message of not being in control, become prime candidates for developing one of the two types of anorexia. Those who refuse to eat are referred to as having the Restricted Type. Those who do eat, sometimes by binging, but then cancel out the calories by vomiting or taking laxatives, are identified as having the Binge-eating/Purging Type (DSM-IV-TR 2000, 589).

Welcome to Madison's world. From her earliest memories she dreamed of being a fashion model. At the ages of six and seven she put on her mother's high heels, draped her big sister's boa around her neck and paraded up and down the hallway between the bedrooms of her house. She imagined she was on a runway with flashing cameras and upbeat music, as she smiled and nodded approval to the wildly accepting audience. Just prior to her eighth birthday, she started begging her mother to enroll her in dance classes that would give her legs the right model curves, and make her look more "refined." It was her most cherished birthday present. Her best friend shared the same career ambition and they played "modeling" during frequent weekend sleep-overs.

For Madison's ninth birthday, her mother took her to a fashion school where she learned about becoming a child model. She sat for her first professional photography session. Every year she received a reward for remaining on the honor roll: an updated professional portfolio. A booking agent for the fashion school secured several jobs for Madison that involved catalog product modeling. Her dream was coming true.

Madison was always self-conscious of how her body looked. Her father teased her about gaining a couple of ounces, not knowing Madison would then forego lunches at school for two or three days to insure those ounces immediately disappeared. By the time she was 12 years old she acted like a dietary expert. She knew the calories, fat content, number of carbs and amount of fiber contained in almost every food item.

As Madison entered puberty, she began gaining weight. Regardless of how she tried to control her diet and increase her work-out routine, she continued to add on a few pounds.

At the same time, her body also grew taller. She was oblivious to the knowledge that the growing bones had weight and it was normal. Madison refused to accept this explanation from her parents and sister. In her mind, all she saw was the weight gain on the bathroom scale—she was getting fat. In two years she had grown five inches. She began to starve herself shortly before her thirteenth birthday.

Madison's mother served her appropriate portions of food for breakfast and dinner, and encouraged snacks between meals. Her father even threatened grounding if she did not eat. Their efforts didn't work and Madison became more desperate. She hated her parents for being angry with her, but wanted to please them. Unfortunately, the fear of gaining weight was much stronger than the desire for pleasing her parents.

A couple months later, Madison attended the next summer modeling school program. She learned from the other girls about using laxatives to "flush out" her system. Madison decided that this was the solution. No one was around to see what Madison ate for breakfast and nobody at school cared whether she ate lunch. At dinner, she ate the food her mother served her and then got rid of it quickly, before her body could absorb it and convert the calories into pounds. This became a nightly activity.

Several months later, Madison's older sister, Erin, walked into their bathroom and caught her. Erin promised not to tell their parents, if Madison agreed to stop taking the laxatives. The agreement lasted for a few months, and in the meantime,

Madison learned about the finger-down-the-throat technique to induce vomiting.

Madison quickly mastered the technique. She learned how to silently throw up, bypassing the normal gag reflex. She used mouthwash twice a day, and always kept a supply of breath mints and strong flavored chewing gum to prevent suspicion of her activities. She fooled everyone, including her sister who assumed Madison was okay. Luckily, the family dentist was knowledgeable about the signs of purging—the enamel on Madison's teeth had begun to erode from constant exposure to stomach acid—and reported her concern.

Alarmed, Madison's mother consulted the family physician. He referred them to a psychiatrist in charge of a residential program that treats eating disorders. Madison checked in to the facility 48 hours later and spent the next several weeks in at the facility. Her father visited her once during her treatment stay. He had a busy work schedule, but passed along his well-wishes through her mother. Erin came two to three times every week, about twice as often as their mother, who attended only one of four scheduled family therapy sessions. It was obvious Madison had little control within her family to gain her parents' support.

Regrettably, Madison was not yet ready to learn about herself. She quickly caught on to the system and played the 'treatment game' well. She deceived the psychiatrist and staff as she temporarily stopped the purging and vomiting behaviors. She said the right things, seemed to genuinely talk about her feelings, and ate small, but consistent meals. She appeared to be making progress.

After slightly more than three weeks, Madison convinced her mother she was well enough to return home. The facility considered her treatment "successful" and discharged her into an aftercare program. She was scheduled to attend group sessions, and see a "recovery counselor" twice a week for the next six months. Five days after discharge she was storing laxatives in her school locker, only bringing one home at a time. Six weeks into the aftercare program, Madison declared herself cured and her parents allowed her to stop seeing the recovery counselor.

Immediately after the family Christmas dinner a few weeks later, Madison purged her food. The old vomiting behavior returned, and went undetected for several additional months. When Madison's face began to look more sunken with darkness under her eyes, Erin became suspicious. She didn't believe Madison's excuse of staying up late studying for exams. She was also aware that her sister had not put tampons on the weekly shopping list for several months. Madison confided to her sister that her menstruation periods had stopped. After Erin shared this information with their mother, Madison's amenorrhea was identified as a symptom of her persisting eating disorder. In coordination with the recovery counselor a family intervention was held.

Madison tearfully admitted to the purging behavior and agreed to fully participate in the treatment program this time. Unfortunately, her father's employer changed health insurance carriers, and the new policy only allowed a fraction of the previous coverage. It would cost the family thousands of dollars for each week of residential treatment and several thousand dollars more for the full aftercare program with follow-up sessions.

The family did not have the resources to cover the cost. Madison's parents also had little confidence that she would remain committed to her recovery work this time, despite her sincerity and tears. Erin offered the remainder of her college savings fund that her parents and grandparents had contributed into for the past ten years. Her parents refused to consider it.

One night, the girls' cousin, Kylie, came to the house to study with Erin for an exam in a college class that they shared. Kylie overheard her aunt and uncle discussing various ways they could possibly afford the costs of Madison's treatment. Optimistically, she shared her experience of being hypnotized as part of a psychology class presentation. Kylie recalled every detail of overcoming her fear of roller coasters with fond memory. She had no idea if this approach would work on an eating disorder, but thought it might be worth investigating.

Kylie shared the presenter's brochure with her aunt. Madison's mother read the material and looked at the website. She still had questions, but the difference in cost certainly made it worth her time to continue checking. She called the family physician and asked about his knowledge of using hypnotherapy to treat eating disorders. He recommended that she call the clinician on the brochure and discuss all of her concerns with him. She called Dr. Lerman's office the next day, and after all of her questions were answered, she scheduled Madison's first appointment.

Madison, now 16 years of age, arrived at the office with her mother and sister. The three of them shared Madison's story. While the individual events were unique to her experience, the historical pattern of obsessive and distorted thinking with compulsive actions was typical of most young people plagued by an eating disorder.

Therapy goals centered on Madison's need to enhance her self-awareness, restore a healthy perception of her body, and build resistance to the negative influences in her environment. Reaching these goals would eliminate her vulnerability and instill self-confidence. These were basically the same goals shared by the psychiatrist at the treatment center. For people like Madison, who are obsessed with the need to be in control, creating a dialog within the mind to problem solve can be a very effective strategy. This is what set hypnosis apart from the traditional treatment program.

There is a specific application in hypnotherapy referred to as "Parts Therapy," in which the unconscious mind is encouraged to establish communication with its several parts. For Madison, these involved her intuition, her creativity, and her imagination. There was also the part which represented the need for control that sustained her anorexic symptoms. Madison assigned a human name to the need for control, "Riley." In her mind it was as if there was another person dictating her choices. At the point when she was ready to detach it from her mind, the release would be like saying goodbye to a negative person. There was no regret or yearning to visit it again.

While in trance Madison allowed the 'all knowing' intuitive part of her mind to communicate with Riley. It secured Riley's agreement to leave her mind when a more effective and less harmful control was identified. She then engaged the creative part of her mind to identify two or three possible solutions that could foster positive control and mastery of her decision-making ability.

The imaginative part was brought in to test how each solution might work, and what consequences they could have. Madison's intuition then selected the best option. At this point Riley's departure was unconditional and expected by her mind. The fear of being fat was replaced by a desire for health and open exploration of different ways to sustain positive self-care. Her mind abandoned the obsession for precision—her new motto was, "progress, not perfection."

A few months later, Madison went in for her semi-annual dental check-up. The dentist found no indication of purging. Over the next year, she gradually gained a total of 26 pounds, bringing her weight to 118 pounds on her five-foot, six-inch frame. After enduring the destructive effects of an eating disorder, Madison ended her modeling career. While completing her college degree, she discovered a creative passion for fashion design. Following her graduation from college, she became a successful clothing designer, styling ensembles that cater to 'average size' young women. She has been free of the anorexia symptoms for more than five years.

For Madison, her shift was ignited by fear. She knew she was out of control and couldn't grasp how that was possible when she was doing everything she could think of to maintain control. Her conscious mind was unable to understand that behavioral control was not the critical control factor. The fear of being fat was the driving energy source for being out of control. There is little logic or rational thinking an adolescent can apply to this level of confusion. As she discovered in trance that she possessed an internal place of control free from fear, she quickly absorbed new learning and began applying it. The knowledge and mastery of her internal strength replaced her sense of fear, allowing the shift in her mind to create permanent change.

CHAPTER 10

Unchartered Waters

The previous client stories in this book reflect typical reasons that bring people in to see a clinical hypnotherapist. The following story began in a similar fashion. Carrie was a 32 year old married woman who initially came in specifically to improve her sex drive. Once she accomplished this, her curiosity turned to a much deeper, extensive desire—to manage the symptoms of her Bi-polar Disorder.

Dr. Lerman thought about the potential treatment plan for such a request, and considered stories of young athletes afflicted with diseases that typically result in permanent disabling conditions. Yet, by refusing to accept these limitations, some athletes are able to overcome the prognoses and exceed medically expected limits. These motivating and inspiring stories convey an important message about the mind's ability to focus healing energy.

Carrie knew Dr. Lerman was a sex therapist, and came to the office for that specific purpose. As he reviewed her intake sheet, he noted that she was under a psychiatrist's care and medicated for Bi-polar Disorder, previously known as "Manic-Depression." This disorder is a result of unstable brain chemistry that causes mood shifts between extreme highs and extreme lows, with rapid drops from the highs to the lows. Irrational behavior and thinking, often triggered by stress or fear, are defining characteristics of manic and depressive episodes (DSM-IV-TR 2000, 382-397).

Carrie began identifying herself as Bi-polar following the experience of her first manic episode at the age of 17. Since that time, her adult life had always been defined by the symptoms of Bi-polar Disorder. Lapses in memory, racing thoughts, or staying up all night working on a jigsaw puzzle were self-labeled as "manic moments." Short periods when she felt no energy, fell asleep shortly after dinner, or had no enthusiasm were parts of her "blah time."

A phone consultation with Carrie's psychiatrist confirmed the Bi-polar diagnosis. He was unaware of the sexual problem, but fully supported her receiving hypnotherapy for it, as well as a more generalized approach to balance her stress level and teach her how to relax. Carrie's third hypnosis session was intended to reinforce the progress made during the first two. However, she stated that passion and enjoyment of sex were becoming everything she had hoped to achieve when she first came to the office. For this session, she asked to shift gears.

Carrie wanted to discover if the same part of her mind which could re-ignite her sexual passion, could also establish a natural mental balance in her brain chemistry. This was uncharted territory for Dr. Lerman, but given his firm belief in the power of the unconscious mind, he was willing and wanting to explore the possibility. Carrie wanted to know if she could prevent the symptoms of her Bi-polar Disorder from happening by using her mind. She clearly understood this was not a typical hypnotherapy application, and that she was free to stop the therapy at any time.

Although Carrie expressed motivation to change the experience of her symptoms, she was still identifying herself as a "Bi-Polar person." Physicians had repeatedly stated that the symptoms were part of a permanent life-time condition. While in the confinement of psychiatric hospitals, Carrie directly witnessed what could happen when patients stopped taking their medications, and lapsed into hypo-manic and psychotic states. With each successive hospitalization, this embedded message evolved into a steadfast belief for what should be expected of her future. Carrie understood that she first had to break through the stigma of a mental illness label.

In order to release the permanence of such a negative image, Carrie had to open her thoughts to the unlimited capacity of her mind. She was presented with a new idea—what if she was not restricted to the boundaries of her history? Carrie began considering what life could be like without Bi-Polar symptoms. The freedom to wonder about other possibilities fueled the power of her imagination. As the unconscious learning process continued each time she went into trance, she felt an awakening of positive energy. The idea of permanent mental illness lost its grip.

Now that Carrie had the creative space to entertain new solutions, she was ready to engage her mind in developing stronger mental skills. In relation to her specific goal, she needed to master the ability to create a flowing awareness of internal messages directing, and redirecting her body's energy.

This kind of complex trance work involves all levels of the mind and requires an enormous amount of concentration by the client. What followed was a series of intensive hypnotherapy sessions, focused on teaching her how to balance the conscious and unconscious parts of her mind.

Carrie did not have an internal frame of reference within which to imagine functioning as a 'normal' adult. Her unconscious mind needed to engage her creativity from the outset of treatment. She controlled the use of her creativity by tapping into the intuitive knowledge stored in her unconscious mind. This intuition held the basis for understanding what healthy, adaptive functioning was like.

Once Carrie discovered the existence of her intuition, she had to learn how it worked. Intuition is a dynamic mental process that goes beyond logic, reasoning, and cognitive thought. It's that message from your gut telling you what to do when logic provides no clue. The sense a mother has when her child is in distress comes from intuition. The same way a person can sense that a loved one has died, despite not being physically present with them.

After gaining a basic understanding of how her intuition worked, Carrie's next task was learning how to rely on it. Her first exercise was locating a reference for normal brain chemistry. She went back in memory, prior to the start of her Bi-polar symptoms. She was very certain that between the ages of 10 and 15 she was happy—no experiences of moodiness or 'dark' thoughts, and behavior very much in sync with a positive self-image. Carrie remembered this period being the last time she truly enjoyed life.

Using her imagination, she took a snapshot of her brain chemistry from her early teens, and transported it into her current mind. Carrie applied the snapshot of healthy chemistry as a template to restructure her current brain functioning. Using an imagined laser beam, she destroyed malformed cells and inserted healthy new ones. The better she became at recognizing bad cells, the easier it was for her to correct faulty chemistry.

In addition to the physical changes in the brain, it was necessary to change the messaging in Carrie's mind. Based on information she shared, Dr. Lerman was able to link positive messages to metaphors woven within a story she could easily relate to. Carrie was fascinated with the Great Pyramids. Prior to a psychotic manic episode, which resulted in another hospitalization that forced her to drop out of school, Egyptian history was her college major.

The metaphor used to reinforce Carrie's emotional stability involved Egyptian Priests who were trained to preserve the bodies of pharaohs and their families after death. The significance of the preservation was to insure each body was kept intact until the soul returned 3,000 years later. Carrie's goal was similar. She was to ensure the continuation of healthy cells and brain chemistry as they were naturally intended—though, 3,000 years may have been a bit more than necessary!

As Carrie became more comfortable trusting her intuition during sessions, she became increasingly proficient with the use of her mind. After learning self-hypnosis, she quickly mastered going into trance on her own to access this knowledge base. She began feeling the excitement of change budding. The message of hope blossomed into her consciousness, along with a new connection to spirituality that she'd never known before. She consistently reported an awareness of healing and feeling healthier, including a state of calmness in her brain. As she continued to exhibit success, the frequency of her visits diminished.

Initially, Carrie's sessions were every day, five days a week for two weeks. Based on reports of her progress, the sessions were reduced to twice a week for two weeks. Then, again, down to one weekly session for six more weeks. Following these intensive sessions, Carrie reported feeling mentally stronger and more focused, with greater internal control. She began attending follow-up appointments on a monthly basis for several months.

It may appear that Carrie's treatment involved a lot of sessions. However, the traditional therapy approach for addressing only the behavioral- and stress-related issues of Bi-polar Disorder can exceed 12 months of weekly sessions. Her treatment took approximately half this time, and began yielding positive changes by the third session.

Carrie was motivated to experience herself without any medications influencing her brain functioning. She went to her next scheduled visit to see her psychiatrist two months after the intensive hypnosis sessions began. She reported the recent positive changes and requested his assistance in weaning her off the prescriptions. The psychiatrist refused her request. He explained that it was not unusual for many Bi-polar patients to experience moments of clarity and believe medications were no longer needed.

Despite disappointment in the psychiatrist's position, Carrie remained determined to discover how well she could function on her own. She explained to her husband that she was going to begin reducing her dosage amounts. She vowed that should she re-experience any signs of the disorder again, she would immediately resume taking the medications. It is important to note that she reached this decision on her own and not at the suggestion or encouragement by anyone else.

Carrie continued her hypnotherapy sessions and listened to the self-hypnosis CD's she received. With the support of her husband, she began weaning herself off of the medications. Despite the gradual reduction in dosage level, she remained able to trust her intuition without hesitation. In addition to this improved emotional balance, Carrie excitedly discovered the return of her memory. Many important events like the births of her two children, and her 10-year wedding anniversary in Hawaii were recalled with vivid detail.

Carrie returned to her psychiatrist for her next scheduled visit three months later. She informed him that since her last appointment, she'd been enjoying her life symptom-free. She related experiencing several stressful events, any one of which could have triggered a manic or depressive reaction. She went on to detail two stories in particular.

The first was an auto accident that resulted when a dump truck made a sharp turn directly in front of her. The truck slammed into her vehicle and totally destroyed the front passenger side. In the past, she would have been paralyzed by fear before lashing out with an over-reactive emotional response, and launching into a hyper-active physical state for several days. Instead, she climbed out of her car and immediately attended to the truck driver to see if he was injured. She dismissed her broken collarbone and superficial cuts as "incidental," but remained very much aware of what could have happened.

Carrie's second story was about her favorite uncle. He suffered a massive stroke that resulted in a comma state. She visited him almost every day for several weeks and left his room in tears each time. She remained at his bedside after the decision was made to stop life support. This type of experience could have plunged her into a deep depression, but she responded very well to the grief of a profound loss, while remaining in control of her feelings.

As Carrie recalled these and other incidents, she impressed the psychiatrist with her recently developed emotional strength and balance. He reluctantly began decreasing her medication dosages without knowing she had already done so. Carrie was absolutely elated! She skipped down the office building steps into the parking lot, and sang with her car radio all the way home. It was a major victory, and she celebrated it with her husband well into the night.

Six months after the start of her therapy, Carrie came in for a follow-up session. She presented herself as a happy, focused, and confident woman. She was now employed at her first job since dropping out of college at the age of 19. She was also in the process of completing her application to resume her college studies. Carrie believed she was in control of her life. Her self-confidence was invigorating!

Carrie comes to the office once a year for her annual 'check-up.' She has been off medications for four years, and remains free of all Bi-polar symptoms. She is a senior in her college studies and will graduate on the dean's list. Her family is planning a trip to visit the Great Pyramids in Egypt in honor of her graduation.

Carrie's journey to change her brain chemistry through the use of hypnosis is most unusual. In theory, whenever the mind causes any change within the body to happen, it is altering the structure of cells in the brain. So the possibility must exist that changing many cells at the same time could alter molecules and bonds which make up the chemistry. Beyond the theory, it was clear that Carrie's curiosity resulted from earlier hypnosis work to restore her sex drive.

The initial success is what signaled her mind to shift into another question of "Why?" She opened her unconscious mind so she could expand her learning beyond what she thought she knew. As the learning happened she realized she was exceptionally more capable than what she originally believed. The path of self-discovery is not concerned with guaranteed results, only the opportunity to explore what is possible.

CHAPTER 11

Childhood Messages

This chapter includes two client stories. Despite the content of each story differing significantly, they are related by a common underlying theme. Neither client realized the profound effect the negative messages their parents gave them as children, had on their adult lives. They needed to first release this messaging before they could resolve the problems plaguing them.

Jerry

In the story about Jerry, golf was prime. He thoroughly enjoyed pleasant days outside, surrounded by exquisite landscaped scenery and the camaraderie of his friends. It was his place to develop business relationships in a social setting. Beyond the coordination and physical skills, golf is a game played between the ears. Jerry liked the mental preparation. However, maintaining focus and emotional balance were critical factors he significantly lacked.

Jerry was 33 years old when he came to Dr. Lerman's office. During the initial interview, he identified himself as a mild-mannered guy in every situation with one exception—when he was on the golf course. It brought out his "dark side." When he made a bad shot, common to every golfer's game, Jerry's inner Hulk emerged and his next few shots reflected his soured mood. He'd slam his clubs down, make sarcastic comments, swear, and carry on as if nobody else on the course existed. Sometimes he competed for small wagers, and when a bad shot cost him a bet, losing made his reactions worse.

Jerry took repeated lessons, practiced more, switched golf clubs, and played different courses. It didn't matter how he tried to change his negative reaction, nothing worked. All he wanted to do was to enjoy playing golf, have more confidence, and feel more in control. "After all," he reasoned, "golf was supposed to be fun and enjoyable." In almost desperation, he arrived at the office hoping that hypnosis could help.

Dr. Lerman introduced a guided imagery technique to keep Jerry focused on his golf game. It included a specific message that regardless of making a good shot or a bad one, once it was done he would release the emotional reaction quietly from his mind. Immediately, he began to focus on his next shot. This is a rather standard post-hypnotic suggestion used with most people wanting to improve their golf game. It is adapted to all other individual sport activities like shooting free throws, hitting or pitching baseballs, throwing footballs, serving in tennis and volleyball, bowling, target shooting, or darts.

The following week, Jerry came in for his second session. He reported feeling more confident and relaxed with far less skepticism about hypnosis. In addition to the guided imagery, he received the suggestion to picture all the negative messages from his past about playing golf on strips of movie film, hanging from a wall in his mind. When he confirmed completing the task, the next suggestion involved him picturing the very best shots he has ever made since he first began playing golf. With each 'best' shot he pointed a finger at one of the film strips and it would drop into a small bottomless hole at the bottom of the wall.

The releasing process continued until all the film strips were gone. The hole then permanently closed. Jerry was asked to play at least two rounds of golf over the next two weeks and use the same finger to point at the ball after each good putt he made. Upon his return to the office, he reported he was having more fun on the golf course and really enjoying the game. His bad temper was almost completely gone and along with it, the previous pressure to make each shot perfect.

Jerry had not previously made the connection between the rejecting messages from his father, RJ, and his flares of anger. The bad golf shots were the common link. He didn't realize that he had never released the anguish from his teenage years. It remained a part of his mind, and he activated it during each round of golf, as soon as made the first bad shot. Once he settled back into trance, he again began putting up the film strips of the negative experiences. This time, an added suggestion included the auditory material to go along with the visual experience. He could hear his father's voice belittling him.

Many of the films involved RJ's harsh, rejecting criticisms while trying to teach Jerry how to play. He was unrelenting in his criticisms of Jerry's grip, his swing, his club selection, his putting stroke, and his opinion of Jerry's overall approach to the game. Jerry absorbed it in, never showing his father the pain or anger he felt. The only place it surfaced was on the golf course away from his father.

Jerry became increasingly agitated as he re-experienced making good putts and pointing his finger at film strips. The first time he did the exercise without hearing sensory memory, there was a far weaker emotional connection. Even though he released many of the negative messages, the direct connection to his father was missing.

Four months later, Jerry sent an email and reported his progress. His handicap improved from 17 to 10. As most golfers know, the best way to lower a handicap is to improve the putting game. That comes from the result of being more relaxed and confident. With each good putt Jerry made, he further reinforced the mental shift from negative to positive messages.

When he came in for a follow-up session, Jerry reported he had invited his dad, RJ, out to play golf with him. He had not played with his father since he was 18 years old to avoid the harsh criticisms. Jerry's perception of RJ had changed. There was a level of tolerance and acceptance not present before, even in situations having nothing to do with golf. He learned to focus on relaxing, concentrating, and allowing only positive energy to flow through him. Jerry's unconscious mind was able to release the negative energy into the hole.

Ellie

Ellie, a 29 year old woman, and her 30 year old husband, Ray, wanted to restore the previous sexual relationship they once enjoyed. From the time they originally met, there was a strong physical attraction and passion. They loved pleasing each other and seemed to lose any prior inhibitions as their relationship developed. A year after marrying they decided to start a family and tried for two years to get pregnant naturally.

The goal to have a child became so dominating they lost sight of their passion for each other, assuming it would remain strong. Their sex life gradually fizzled out with the mounting frustration and breakdown in their intimacy.

Even though the couple desired to have a child, no matter how often they had sex or when in her menstruation cycle they did, Ellie could not become pregnant. Frustrated with their inability to begin a family, Ellie and Ray turned to costly medical procedures. The first fertility specialist they saw collected several vials of blood, a filled urine cup, vaginal and uterine tissues samples, and eggs for lab analysis on Ellie. Ray was sent down the hall to see the urologist for a physical exam and asked to leave a sperm sample for analysis.

A week later they returned and received the results of the lab work. There were no identified medical problems. They felt relieved hearing they were healthy, but still confused as to why Ellie had not been able to get pregnant. The doctor indicated that the initial lab work was only part of a number of tests they would consider.

Over the next several weeks, Ellie and Ray followed the doctor's orders about when, and in what positions to have sexual intercourse. They then progressed to the harvesting process of her eggs. He continued depositing his sperm at regular weekly visits so her harvested eggs could be inseminated. For Ray, masturbating in the tiny clinic room became increasingly distasteful and stressful. All the fun and excitement of spontaneous love-making disappeared.

They were told not to have sex for several weeks while the in-vitro process of placing fertilized eggs in her uterus occurred. Ellie and Ray were both avid movie goers, but stopped going to avoid getting aroused from watching a sexy scene. For this same reason, they also stopped having romantic dinners. Even snuggling on the couch and reading, or watching television became uncomfortable.

Further adding to the discomfort was the financial end of trying to get pregnant. The total cost of all the treatments was well in excess of $120,000. Their health insurance paid for none of it. They borrowed from both sets of parents, and it would have all been worth it to them, if there was a reasonable likelihood of a healthy pregnancy. Based on the results obtained to that point, the doctors could not offer any percent of possible success. They were never able to identify a specific reason why the fertilization process did not work, so other than continuously repeating the same procedures with minor tweaks, there was no confidence of a positive outcome. They even briefly toyed with the idea of using an agency to find a woman with similar DNA to Ellie's, and having Ray's sperm artificially inserted to impregnate her.

Although Ellie's OB/GYN suggested they continue to harvest and freeze eggs for later fertilization, the couple was moving into a belief of hopelessness. After six years of negative clinical intervention, Ellie and Ray struggled and argued with each other. Coming to grips with accepting that producing a child naturally, or by artificial means was not likely to happen yielded a deeply felt emptiness.

The entire process became so clinical and emotionally detached that Ellie and Ray had unintentionally distanced themselves from each other. They were burned out, and coupled with their feelings of defeat, lost their individual sexual desire and mutual attraction. They loved each other and wanted help to reconnect on a passionate level.

During the next session, Ellie and Ray agreed to share the experience of hypnosis together. Several different exercises intended to connect their energy yielded a very positive reaction. These exercises are only possible when both partners are completely focused. They sensed and felt the flow of their own inner energy fields, the Qi.

Ellie and Ray then learned to experience each other's Qi, as they practiced exchanging and intertwining their energy. They worked on touching and holding exercises intended to communicate the desire to share passion. The homework assignments included sharing more non-verbal physical messages to each other of love, sensuality, seduction and sexual touching. They learned a self-hypnosis technique that focused on directing the Qi to flow into their erogenous zones and sexual organs. At the start of the third session, they reported a rediscovery of their sexual energy and passion for each other, along with the fun and silliness of being together. It was very similar to the infatuation and "puppy love" they shared during the start of their relationship.

At the end of the third session, Ellie asked if it was possible for her to experience in trance what it would be like for one of her eggs to become fertilized. She had no difficulty imagining having a child, but the process of fertilization and pregnancy were never clear images. Over the next two sessions, Ellie worked on releasing negative messages acquired during adolescence about pregnancy and the damaged social reputation that comes from becoming sexually active. These sessions were critically important.

During her early adolescent years, Ellie received a constant assault of messages from her parents, mostly her mother. They were intended to suppress natural curiosity and scare Ellie away from all sexual activity. Her parents obsessively worried about her becoming promiscuous. They had dreams and aspirations for her and did not want her to accidentally become pregnant, or so absorbed in boys that she would decrease attention from her school work and violin lessons.

There is often a fine line between parents acting in the best interest of their children, by enforcing unyielding standards, and acting out their own unfulfilled dreams, by imposing them onto their children. Sometimes there are cultural influences that parents were raised to maintain and pass down to the next generation. Well intentioned or not, these negative messages became internalized by Ellie. The most powerful message of all foreshadowed what would become a near disastrous ironic twist—"Do not become pregnant. It will ruin your life."

Ellie was not aware these messages could affect her biology. This is not unusual. Most people have little awareness of the mind/body connection, particularly concerning sexuality. Clients are frequently referred to recommended materials to learn about sexual biology. Dr. Christina Northrup's book, Women's Bodies, Women's Wisdom (2010) is particularly useful for young women.

Once Ellie consciously understood the powerful impact the negative messaging had on her life, the next step was to teach her how to let it go. While in trance she learned how to activate the intuitive and imaginative parts of the unconscious mind. She could picture herself standing inside of an igloo-like room. On the walls were small strips of paper that contained all the negative messages she had received during her life, as well as all the positive messages. She learned she could remove the negative messages and caste them out, so they would never affect her again. At the same time she learned to embrace all the positive messages and to reflect upon those messages whenever an important decision was needed.

Ellie then applied her imagination to her biology and reproductive system. She began experiencing what it would be like to feel her eggs as they flowed down during ovulation, became fertilized, and nestled into her uterus during pregnancy. The final step of this imagination process involved the birthing and delivery of her born child. Between sessions, she practiced self-hypnosis every day, and charted her daily body temperature to determine the course of her menstruation cycle.

Ellie and Ray became more passionate and romantic as their love making fulfilled their initial expectations. Their mutual desire and satisfaction exceeded what they first experienced several years before. The obsession and frustration about fertilization was gone. Even with Ellie taking her temperature every morning and practicing self-hypnosis, she was calm and relaxed.

The next follow-up sessions were scheduled to coincide with Ellie's next two ovulation periods. Following the same guided imagery previously done, these sessions focused on the natural biological workings of her body. Three months later Ray called reporting Ellie was pregnant. She then came in once a month and continued to receive post-hypnotic suggestions reinforcing the normal biology of pregnancy.

As Ellie entered her seventh month of pregnancy the trance work shifted to the birthing process and reinforcing her positive expectations. She and Ray attended natural childbirth classes and at full-term, Ellie delivered a healthy seven pound baby girl without any anesthesia or pain medication. There was no tearing and no need for an episiotomy. Ellie and Ray left the hospital the next day proud parents, eagerly looking forward to their future family life together.

Prior to and subsequent to the work done with Ellie and Ray, there were referrals from OB/GYN's requesting assistance in helping women experience sexual desire. However, there were never any physician referrals related to fertility. Those only originated from couples, always after spending tens of thousands, sometimes over one hundred thousand dollars. All of the couples had experienced many failures, and repeated cycles of hope, followed by despair. When the brain is free to work, it is the most powerful sexual organ in the human body.

So, what do Jerry and Ellie have in common? Both Jerry and Ellie received powerful parental messages that became imbedded in their minds during adolescence. For Jerry, the message was simple, "You are a failure unless you play golf as I tell you." For Ellie, it was equally simple, "Do not get pregnant or your life will be worthless." Jerry became an irritable and angry golfer, who beat himself up when he made a bad shot or didn't win the friendly wager. Ellie internalized the message to such a degree her eggs would not progress through fertilization, even when fertilized outside of her body, placed in her uterus and then subsequently into the uterus of another woman. Once these two people released the negative messages, they fulfilled their expectations.

The process of seeking help involving hypnosis quite often starts with a known problem or issue, and then opens into an experience far beyond what the surface, conscious mind understood. Allowing access into the unconscious mind with a specific intention is quite often the initiation to a special discovery. It becomes a new learning, clearly establishing the awareness that we know so much more than we think we do.

CHAPTER 12

Unintended Benefits

Sometimes it is very simple to discover the "why" prompting a client who wants to change a behavior, stop a bad habit, or release negative messages. Sometimes it isn't necessary for the hypnotherapist to know why, as long as the client accomplishes his or her reason for receiving the help. One of the more fascinating aspects of working with people in trance is that they often experience unintended benefits, along with the identified goal. This provides an even greater appreciation for the amazing power of the mind to generalize healing messages and suggestions. It also further supports the awareness of how the unconscious part of the mind is able to go beyond consciousness in applying healing where it is needed. The following short client stories are all presentations of unintended benefits.

Norma

Norma was a 44 year old woman when she arrived for her appointment. She appeared healthy, and although somewhat overweight, there was no mention of weight being a concern. Her goal was to stop smoking. Except for brief periods of time when pregnant with her children, she was a smoker for 29 years. Her decision to stop resulted from the pledge she made the last time she saw her mother alive, the evening prior to her death from lung cancer.

Norma easily went into a hypnotic trance, and after the second session, reported she no longer had the desire to smoke. 30 days later she reported remaining free from cigarettes. After four months Norma proudly affirmed she was a non-smoker. She then asked rather inquisitively if she received a post-hypnotic suggestion regarding weight loss. She was losing weight at the rate of almost two pounds a week.

This was very confusing to Norma. All her adult life she heard nasty stories of people gaining weight after they stopped smoking. This was her conscious concern. Part of her hesitancy for many years about quitting was the dreaded weight gain. Norma received only one post-hypnotic suggestion specifically related to food: she would not feel the need to eat as a substitute for smoking, because of her commitment to becoming healthy in every way. There were no suggestions about losing weight.

Several months later she sent in an unsolicited testimonial email. She proudly proclaimed passing the one year mark as a non-smoker, as well as being 28 pounds lighter. Norma then described an additional positive result. She was no longer smoking marijuana. She never identified doing this during the sessions. She viewed this type of smoking as a purely occasional activity and did not consciously consider it a cause for treatment.

Norma smoked marijuana with her sorority sisters while in college, and continued afterwards when they would get together about once a month. The ladies smoked the last time they met, but Norma passed and never took a "hit." She simply had no desire to engage, and was surprised she did so without a second thought.

The post-hypnotic suggestions about becoming "smoke-free," and "healthy in every way," embedded themselves in her unconscious mind. The creative part of her mind identified solutions for how this could happen and then her intuition transformed the solutions into decisions restoring her to balance and harmony.

Kelly

At the time of treatment, Kelly was a 38 year old woman and the mother of two teenagers. She came to the office specifically wanting to stop having panic attacks in reaction to freeway driving. Travelling that fast, particularly on the elevated sections, terrified her. The fear was so intense she was unable to sleep the night before having to drive downtown, or take her daughter to cheerleading camp on the other side of town during the summer. Her desperation became so great that she would only drive on surface roads. Repeatedly, she would call her husband to get the "safest" directions, and then call her brother to confirm her husband's information.

Kelly knew that her fear created inconvenience, wasted time and often resulted in her being late—which only compounded her stress level. For the past three years her physician prescribed various dosage levels of anti-depressants and the anti-anxiety medication, Xanax. The relief was minimal, but she was afraid to not take the pills, believing her panic might escalate. When she received a summons for jury duty, she became extremely fearful of what awaited her. Driving to the courthouse would require elevated freeway driving and some of it was over water, another panic trigger.

Kelly's sister-in-law had used hypnosis and became a non-smoker four years earlier. She tried many times to convince Kelly to get help, and even offered to drive her. Kelly shrugged it off because she didn't understand hypnosis, and changing any routine or thought process was hard.

Eventually, Kelly's need to overcome the fear was greater than not doing anything. When she arrived for her initial appointment, Kelly had no idea what to expect. She was extremely nervous and expressed serious doubts about the entire process. She didn't think she could be hypnotized because she always had to be in control. She laughed in response to the observation of how she "controlled" her fear of freeway driving. As overly rational and logical people try to defend against changing, there is one inevitable truth that always seems to emerge: fears and phobias are not logical or rational. They are created and empowered by emotional reaction.

Kelly agreed to "try" and relax after receiving assurances that it was her choice as to when she would relax, and when she would to go into a hypnotic trance. The reality of why people seek help is based on motivation to stop doing or thinking something unwanted, or to learn something important about themselves. The initial resistance is simply the scariness of letting go.

As Kelly followed directions for breathing deeply and releasing tension, she maintained finger movements and flexed her left ankle every few seconds. Sometimes this can be an involuntary action for people with various kinds of neuro-muscular illnesses like cerebral palsy, Parkinson's disease, Attention Deficit/Hyperactivity Disorder, or head trauma injuries (American Association of Neurological Surgeons 2005). For these people, the movement does not interfere with the trance induction or the positive gains that the unconscious mind can generate. However, when these kinds of movements are utilized by people attempting to remain conscious, it is counterproductive to the therapy.

The easiest way to determine if body movements are intentional is to implode the message of control. This is an Ericksonian technique designed to overload the conscious mind with confusion until it releases control to the subconscious mind. Kelly received permission to continue with these movements. At the same time she received another suggestion that she might find it interesting to see what would happen if she alternated moving the fingers on one hand, while keeping the fingers on the other hand still, then moving the fingers on the other hand while keeping the original moving fingers still. Another suggestion followed indicating she might find it interesting to see what might happen if she flexed her left ankle after the second time she moved the right ring finger, then the

6th time and the 26th time. Then after the 33rd time she might find it interesting if the fingers on her right hand did not want to move anymore.

Kelly kept following the suggestions of moving one specific finger on her left hand, followed by flexing the ankle after an arbitrary number. The desired confusion took effect after a very short time. Then she received the imploding suggestion which indicated that she might find it interesting for all of her fingers to simply decide to rest comfortably, as her ankle rested too. Within four or five seconds of receiving the last suggestion, her conscious mind let go. All movement stopped and she drifted comfortably into trance.

Kelly became noticeably calmer. While in trance she went back in time and identified witnessing two frightening car wrecks on the freeway. In addition, there was one episode of her hydroplaning and losing control of her car on an overpass. By the end of the third session she reported successfully detaching the fearful emotions from the events by using the same trauma releasing technique used with people who have PTSD. The panic attacks were gone. She did not experience any more sleepless nights or irritability, and no longer sought alternate routes to avoid freeway driving.

Kelly returned to the office two months later for a follow-up session. This time her two children accompanied her. Her fifteen year old daughter, Amanda, and thirteen year old son, Eric, wanted to talk in private in their own session. Kelly shrugged her shoulders and agreed. Amanda and Eric disclosed being absolutely thrilled with their mother's progress. Both were curious about the process she went through, and how they could potentially benefit from using hypnosis.

Amanda went on to describe how her mother had developed a rather nasty habit of hovering over her while she did her homework, practiced piano or talked to anybody on the phone. Kelly also lectured her daughter incessantly, making sure she heard all the possible bad consequences to almost every decision she made. Amanda hated it, but no amount of begging, pleading or reasoning would make Kelly stop.

The calmness now in Kelly was remarkable, and Amanda wanted to share her thanks for the improvement in her relationship with Kelly. Eric jokingly asked if his mother was on a "magic pill." Kelly was no longer dropping him off for choir practice, and was no longer worrying about "every little thing." He reported they laughed a lot more, even while driving to the store or across town.

At no time during the sessions with Kelly were the issues of her hovering, lecturing or habitual lateness ever addressed. The unconscious mind facilitated the healing process and released the fear of driving. The internal value for calmness generalized into those areas of Kelly's mind previously absorbed by negative energy. As she created a positive frame of reference, potentially stressful events became easily manageable. The resulting confidence spread to Amanda and Eric.

Children learn from their parents through role modeling, and just like high-priced paper toweling, they absorb it all—the good, the bad, and the ugly. Amanda mentioned that her best friend told her to stop being so bossy and telling her what to do. She wondered if maybe that was the reason boys didn't show her much attention. As much as she hated being on the receiving end of it from her mother, she had learned it, and was unintentionally repeating the behavior.

Eric complained about having to serve another detention in school for tardiness. Seems he just could not get to class on time. His choir teacher threatened to cancel his solo performance at the spring concert, if he was late one more time. Both children requested hypnosis sessions to eliminate these learned behaviors. It took them one session each to make the desired changes. Their expectation to change was locked in place from witnessing and taking part in Kelly's success.

Albert

Albert's story is a classic example of a very smart young man caught in the vortex of social anxiety. When he arrived at the office for his initial visit, he provided an unsolicited written autobiography including a history of always being very self-conscious. He never had more than one friend at a time, no history of dating, and no confidence in standing up for himself or his ideas.

At 29 years of age, Albert achieved seven years of exemplary work history with the same company. He had recently learned that a promotion he assumed would be his went to someone else for the second time. He resentfully explained the promotion snub was political because he was not one of the "good old boys." He did not understand how his repeated absences from the annual Christmas party and other company sponsored social functions, created a negative impression or had anything to do with an evaluation for promotion.

There is more to realizing success in business than just possessing intelligence, ambition and productivity. Senior management often looks at other traits when evaluating and recommending employees for promotion. Most often these traits include leadership, confidence and social skills. For those talented and very smart young professionals who lack these non-performance skills, the result of diminished recognition and missed opportunities for promotion are very frustrating.

Albert's disdain for social interaction was interpreted by superiors as poor leadership potential. Quite often, deficits in social skills and lacking confidence are signs of social anxiety. He was unusually withdrawn, very self-conscious and not confident beyond his specific areas of technical expertise. These factors are very typical of people experiencing this type of anxiety.

The youngest of three brothers, Albert experienced chronic teasing and verbal put-downs throughout childhood by his brothers. As he got older, the teasing extended to neighborhood children and schoolmates. Sticks and stones can hurt you—and words can hurt even more.

Albert responded by avoiding social contact and retreating into a solitary life while mastering academics. Throughout his academic years, his love for math and science led him to excel in these classes, and earned a full academic scholarship to a private university in Houston. Graduating with high honors in chemistry and a minor in mathematics, he received numerous job offers from all over the world. He chose the position of a chemical analyst at a local petroleum company. He wanted to remain within the certainty of knowing his surroundings.

Albert was into his eighth year with the same company. Despite creating three process patents and having several articles published in leading trade journals, he could not get promoted. The only person he could confide in was his one friend, Gina. They originally met as lab partners in a college freshman chemistry class. She was late for the first day of class and the only unoccupied seat was next to Albert. For the first half of the semester the only words exchanged between them concerned the chemistry experiments shared in lab. They were the only two in class to score a perfect 100 percent on the midterm exam, and she invited him to celebrate at a local pizza place.

Albert respected Gina as she possessed a similar brilliance in chemistry. Over the years their talks broadened to other topics and they became good friends. She clearly was not a girlfriend in any romantic sense, although he did admit to occasionally wondering what she looked like without any clothes on. He could not allow himself to think about her in any sexual way for fear of losing her friendship. She was, however, extremely perceptive and seemed to intuitively know what Albert was feeling better than Albert did.

Clearly, Gina similarly valued their friendship and if she had any romantic feelings for him, they remained well hidden. She made sure when they were in her apartment to always remain fully clothed, even when unwinding from a finished project or completed final exams. She suggested he talk with someone knowledgeable in neuro-linguistic programming (NLP) to see if he could learn how to stop feeling so self-conscious and act more like his co-workers.

Gina learned about NLP while in college to overcome a problem with test anxiety. Due to the strong research base for linguistic patterns, she found it academically sound and could recommend it to Albert. NLP is a therapy process that originated from Erickson's teachings and developed into a specific therapy style in the 1970s (Andreas and Faulkner 1994, 27). It focuses on the internalized meaning of words. The process is a learning approach in which clients change their use of words, and word patterns, to effect changes in awareness and behavior.

Upon arrival for an initial appointment at Dr. Lerman's office, Albert's anxiety was obvious. He sat very rigid, made minimal eye contact, and kept glancing at his watch. He managed to explain his problem, but had a near impossible time using his imagination to describe how he would be different once the problem was gone. Establishing a positive rapport is a critical necessity for any type of therapy effectiveness. Considering how restricted Albert was in talking about himself, an indirect approach seemed like the best strategy to open up communication.

Dr. Lerman asked Albert if he was familiar with the Prisoner's Dilemma. It is a non-competitive mental game created by Anatol Rapoport, a mathematician, psychologist, philosopher, music composer, and noted genius in several fields. His teachings are presented in advanced college mathematics courses throughout North America and Europe. Albert reported studying the game for hours as a college student. He found it so intriguing he would actually solicit other students to engage in the game. Dr. Lerman asked him to remember what he first learned about the game and to describe what he experienced. Albert quickly became more animated as he spoke for several minutes. They then talked about the value of cooperation and communication. As he began relaxing, he could imagine sitting in front of Dr. Rapoport and talking with him about the game.

At this point Albert was completely free in his expression, and even made a few hand gestures as he spoke. He could easily identify with the word connections of being like a prisoner, trapped within his mind. The game presented an interesting possibility, beyond its intention. Albert now understood a way out of his dilemma. He could imagine relating to the needs for cooperation and communication. He began looking at his social life as a series of choices. Each choice could be seen as a dilemma to which he could select the best solution.

Albert had two additional sessions. Each started with a review of the various "dilemmas" he solved during the week. His choice of words became more proactive and intentional. As the self-consciousness diminished he became increasingly more confident. His use of language became freer and his expressed understanding of others created a level of connection he found appealing and accepting by others.

Over the next several months, Albert continued practicing until he became so confident of his new communication style that it became automatic. Albert released himself from the imprisoned life he knew. He unintentionally discovered a link to a passion for communication. He became active with a national association of professional chemists, presenting research papers on his work, and broader topics like ethics and philosophy.

Originally seeking assistance for overcoming social anxiety in order to move his career forward, Albert opened his mind. He learned to communicate effectively, relate to people better, and let go of self-consciousness. The unintended benefit of realizing his passion allowed him to take emotional risks by sharing his thoughts with others. His career was fully developing, as was his life in many directions. Several months later during a follow-up phone call, Albert reported he and Gina were now "an item." His curiosity of what she looked like without clothes was probably resolved.

Our ability to exceed what we consciously know about ourselves is unlimited. The commitment to become healthy in one aspect is generalized to others. The confidence of overcoming a specific fear is applied to other anxiety-invoking issues. The elimination of social awkwardness includes resolving many interactive problems. These are clear examples of what our minds can do once they are opened and actively working while in trance.

Norma, Kelly and Albert thought they knew what they needed to know about themselves. They were settling for less than what each was capable of experiencing. Once they discovered that they knew much more, the excitement of positive change created a momentum of flowing energy. Their minds shifted into a direction of anticipated success, satisfaction, and happiness as the motion of their lives began moving forward.

CHAPTER 13

Conclusion

The inspiration for this book comes from the successful outcomes of thousands of clients who have learned to experience the healing ability of the unconscious mind through the use of hypnosis. The case stories presented are a very small sample of people who demonstrated positive changes from a multitude of presenting problems.

The intent of the book is to illustrate the amazing ability of the unconscious mind to create positive change and healing. Throughout childhood and during adulthood, we are trained to learn and value cognitive skills. The ability to think, use logic, derive rational expectations, and sound conclusions, are valuable and essential aspects of how we function and gain knowledge from the outside world. However, these skills only represent a small portion our minds. They do not define who we are as human beings or our potential.

The vast majority of the mind contains our inner strength. It incorporates imagination, creativity, intuitive understanding, feelings, memory and biology, while balancing our thoughts and feelings. Hypnosis is the most effective tool for activating all parts of the mind. The messages received while in trance are intended to focus the unconscious mind to a specific topic or issue. The internal energy connects every aspect of the mind to facilitate understandings, learning, solutions, changes, and resolution.

For all the attention recently generated by the growing acceptance of how our minds and bodies are connected, these are not new concepts. They simply became more popular. Similarly, we have known for decades about stress and how it can manifest into physical and mental illnesses. At the same time, the practices of medical care and mental health are shifting from healing people to focusing on treating symptoms. Unfortunately, reactions to stress are far too often considered only in terms of symptoms. Treating them with medications and advice about exercising, eating better and cutting down on alcohol, may help to temporarily manage the reactions, but fails to provide permanent change.

At a logical level of understanding, we know it is not possible for the mind and body to experience tension and relaxation at the same time. We know the mind and body work far less efficiently when stressed. We know the most effective way to concentrate and problem solve is with a calm, uncluttered mind. We know the best method for increasing worker productivity is by decreasing tension and pressure. We know one of the first words out the mouths of parents, teachers, and coaches when encountering an emotionally upset child is, "relax."

We live in a world of tension and conflict. Yet we also have the ability within ourselves to maintain balance and harmony. One of the goals in writing this book is to demonstrate how we can experience life with meaning, value, and purpose by learning how to go inside our minds, and activate the natural healing energy we possess. We are fully capable of living our lives in balance with the natural connection between our minds and our bodies. The examples presented in the chapters represent a few situations for which hypnosis has successfully ignited substantial healthy life-long change.

There is now an abundance of clinical hypnosis research reflecting positive changes in people's lives. It includes the areas of emotional release, improved health, pain reduction, professional and business success, sports improvement, overcoming fears and anxiety, sexual performance, self-improvement, academic success, attitude changes, letting go of bad relationships, and stopping unhealthy habits.

One of the most frequently heard comments when clients complete their hypnotherapy program is, "Why don't more people know about this?" The answer is simply that as clinicians we do not have vast resources to invest in advertising and promotions. Our educational process of reaching others comes from the clients we help, or people reading magazine articles, or watching television programs presenting honest information. We expect the readers of this book will generate more discussion and further inquiry, perhaps to satisfy their curiosity by experiencing hypnosis first hand. Imagine what could be better about your life once your unconscious mind shifts beyond what you think you know.

ABOUT THE AUTHORS

Marty Lerman received his Ph.D. in Educational Psychology from the University of Wisconsin-Milwaukee. Ten years later he was running a successful mental health private practice and teaching psychology and counseling courses at area colleges and universities. He also completed post-graduate training to gain certifications as a sex therapist, medical psychotherapist and palliative care specialist. He received his initial training in hypnosis and hypnotherapy at the Ericksonian Institute in Houston, Texas.

Under the instruction of Drs. Carol Kershaw and Bill Wade, he acquired extensive knowledge of Ericksonian philosophy, therapy techniques, and trance application. There followed years of additional courses and readings which led to a deeper appreciation for the unconscious mind and the inner energy we possess. For the past twenty years he has fully integrated trance work and hypnotherapy into his clinical practice.

Samuel Kupper earned his Ph.D. from the University of Michigan in the field of Chinese History and Philosophy. He also has a law degree from Loyola Law School in Los Angeles and is a member of the California State Bar. Among his numerous fellowships, he is the recipient of a Fulbright Fellowship, and those from both the American Council of Learned Societies and the Social Science Research Council. In his younger years, he practiced self-hypnosis with incredible success. Upon retiring, he sought to explore the possibility of using hypnosis and self-hypnosis as a means of gaining greater understanding and utilization of his inner energy field.

RESOURCES

For more information about Dr. Lerman and the services available from his clinic, please visit either website at www.Facebook.com/AlliedHypnosis or www.AlliedHypnosis.com.

For more information about practicing certified and consulting hypnotists, please visit the National Guild of Hypnotists website at www.ngh.net

For more information about the Milton H. Erickson Institute and trained clinicians, please visit the American Society of Clinical Hypnosis website: www.asch.net.

The following is a partial list of stress reactors and other conditions that can be successfully helped with hypnosis:

Mind and body relaxation

Sleep better

Weight control

Stop smoking

Pain relief

Headache release

Improve memory

Better concentration

Improve focus

Test taking fear

Improved study habits

Confidence gain

Stop procrastinating

Public speaking fear

More intuitive

Letting go of habits

Erase bad labels

Anger control

Release guilt

Forgiveness

Grieving and loss

Improve sex desire

Stop teeth grinding

Stop hair pulling

Improve gag reflex

Fear of needles

Bad eating habits
Medical/Dental fear
Childbirth pain
Skin disorders
More assertive
Better sales prep
Over-worrying
Stage fright
Fingernail biting
Goal setting
Sports improvement
Releasing past hurts
Inner control
Organization skills

REFERENCES

American Association of Neurological Surgeons. *Movement Disorders.* September 2005. Accessed September 13, 2012. http://www.aans.org/PatientInformation/Conditionand Treatments/MovementDisorders.aspx.

Andreas, Steve and Charles Faulkner, eds. *NLP: The New Technology of Achievement.* New York: William Morrow and Company, 1994.

Bowen, Alison. "PTSD Reports Increase Among 9/11 Responders," *New York Times, Metro,* 10/13/2011. Accessed September 13, 2012. www.metro.us/newyork/local/article/996525.

Breggin, Peter R. *Talking Back to Ritalin: What Doctors Aren't Telling You About Stimulants and ADHD.* Cambridge, MA: DaCapo Press, 2001.

Breggin, Peter R. *Brain Disabling Treatments in Psychiatry: Drugs, Electroshock, and the Psychopharmaceutical Complex.* New York: Springer Publishing, 2008.

Charach, Alice and Others. "Attention Deficit Hyperactivity Disorder: Effectiveness of Treatment in At-Risk Preschoolers; Long-term Effectiveness in All Ages; and Viability in Prevalence, Diagnosis, and Treatment." *Comparative Effectiveness Review No. 44.* Prepared by the McMaster University Evidence-based Practice Center under Contract

No. MME 2202 290-02-0020. AHRQ Publication No. 12-EHC003-EF. Rockville, MD: Agency for Healthcare Research and Quality, U.S. Department of Health and Human Services. October 2011.

Cousins, Norman. *Anatomy of an Illness As Perceived By the Patient: Reflections on Healing and Regeneration.* New York: W. W. Norton and Company, 1979.

Diagnostic and Statistical Manual of Mental Disorders, Fourth Edition, Text Revision. Washington, DC: American Psychiatric Association, 2000.

Einstein, Albert. *Ideas and Opinions.* New York: Random House, 1954.

Elder, T and Others. "The Importance of Relative Standards in ADHD Diagnosis: Evidence Based on Exact Birth Dates." *Journal of Health Economics* 29, no. 5 (2010): 641-656.

Gallagher, Barry B. *The Secrets of Life Power: How to Open the Door to Your Best Life.* Mequon, WI: Nightengale Press, 2008.

Hagerty, Rebecca G. and Others. "Communicating Prognosis in Cancer Care: a Systemic Review of the Literature." *Annals of Oncology* 17, no. 7 (2005): 1005-1053.

Hartsell, William F. and Others. "Can Physicians Accurately Predict Survival Time in Patients Metastic Cancer? Analysis of

RTOG97-14." *Journal of Palliative Medicine* 11, no. 5 (2008): 723-728.

Jensen, Peter S., and Others. "3-Year Follow-up of the NIMH MTA Study." *Journal of the American Academy of Child & Adolescent Psychiatry* 46, no. 8 (2007): 989-1002.

Jung, Carl G. *Collective Works of C. G. Jung, Vol. 9, Part 2. 2nd Edition.* Princeton, NJ: Princeton University Press, 1968.

Lamont, Elizabeth B. and Nicholas A. Christakis. "Prognostic Disclosure to Patients with Cancer Near the End of Life." *Annals of Internal Medicine* 134, no. 12 (2001): 1096-1105.

Lankton, Stephen R. and Carol H. Lankton. *The Answer Within: A Clinical Framework of Ericksonian Hypnotherapy.* New York: Brunner/Mazel, 1983.

Levin, Harvey S. "Neuroplasticity and Brain Imaging Research: Implications for Rehabilitation." *Archives of Physical Medicine and Rehabilitation.* 87, no. 12 Supplement 2 (2006): S1.

Lobliner, Jill and Courtney Rees. "New Study Shows Early Ritalin May Cause Long-term Effects on Brain." *Medical News Today,* December 13, 2004. Accessed September 13, 2012. http://www.medicalnewstoday.com/releases/17691.php.

McKeown, Robert. University of South Carolina. "Attention Deficit Hyperactivity Disorder is Both Under and Over Diagnosed Study Suggests." *Science Daily,* October 19, 2012.

Accessed November 30, 2012. http://www.sciencedaily/releases/2012/10/12109141124.htm.

Northrup, Christiane. *Women's Bodies, Women's Wisdom: Creating Physical and Emotional Health and Healing*. New York: Random House, 2010.

Ochs, Ridgely. "9/11 First Responders" Battle With PTSD." *Newsday,* August 18, 2011. Accessed July 16, 2012. http://www.newsday.com/911-anniversary/9-11-first-responders-battle-with-ptsd-1.3107122.

Oregon Health & Science University. "Drug Effectiveness Review Project, ADHD Medications, Final Report." *The OHSU Drug Effectiveness Review,* December, 2011. Accessed August 4, 2012. http://www.ohsu.edu/drugeffectiveness.

Ranchaud, R., Schell, T.L., Karney, B.R., Osilla, K.C., Burns, R.M, Caldarone, L.B. "Disparate Prevalence Estimates of PTSD Among Service Members Who Served in Iraq and Afghanistan: Possible Explanations." *Journal of Traumatic Stress* 23, no. 1 (2010): 59-68.

Reston, James. *Special to The New York Times*. "Now, About My Operation in Peking." *New York Times (1857-current file),* ProQuest Historical Newspapers The New York Times (1951-2004). Accessed January 3, 2013. http://www.graphics8.nytimes.com/packages/pdf/health/1971acupuncture.pdf.

Roan, Shari. "Women on War Front More Likely to Get Post-traumatic Stress Disorder Than Men, Study Finds." *Los Angeles Times, Local,* May 19, 2011. Accessed October 14, 2012. http://www.articles.latimes.com/2011/may/19/news/la-heb-ptsd-women-military-20110519.

Standifer, Cid. "PTSD Diagnostic Rates Rise Among Female Troops." *Army Times,* March 12, 2012. Accessed October 14, 2012. http://www.armytimes.com/news/2012/03/military-times-20120poll-ptsd-diagnostic-rates-rise-female-troups-031212w/.

Star Wars Episode IV: A New Hope, Film, Directed by George Lucas. 1977. Los Angeles, CA: 20th Century Fox.

Sugrue, Thomas. *There Is a River, 75th Anniversary Edition.* New York: Dell Publishing, 1976.

Tourneur, Maurice, Director. *Trilby.* Fort Lee, NJ: World Film Company, 1923.

Walker, Sidney III. *The Hyperactivity Hoax: How to Stop Drugging Your Child and find Real Medical Help.* New York: St. Martin's Press. 1998.

White, Erin. Northwestern University. "Diagnosis of ADHD on the Rise." *Science Daily,* March 19, 2012. Accessed August 4, 2012. http://www.sciencedaily.com/releases/2012/03/120319134214.htm

Wilson, C. Philip, ed. *Fear of Being Fat: The Treatment of Anorexia Nervosa and Bulimia, Revised Edition.* Northvale, NJ: Jason Aronson, 1987.

Wolraich, Mark and Others. "Clinical Practice Guidelines for the Diagnosis, Evaluation, and Treatment of Attention-deficit/ Hyperactivity Disorder in Children and Adolescents." *Pediatrics* 128, no. 5 (2011): 1007-1022.

starborn
support